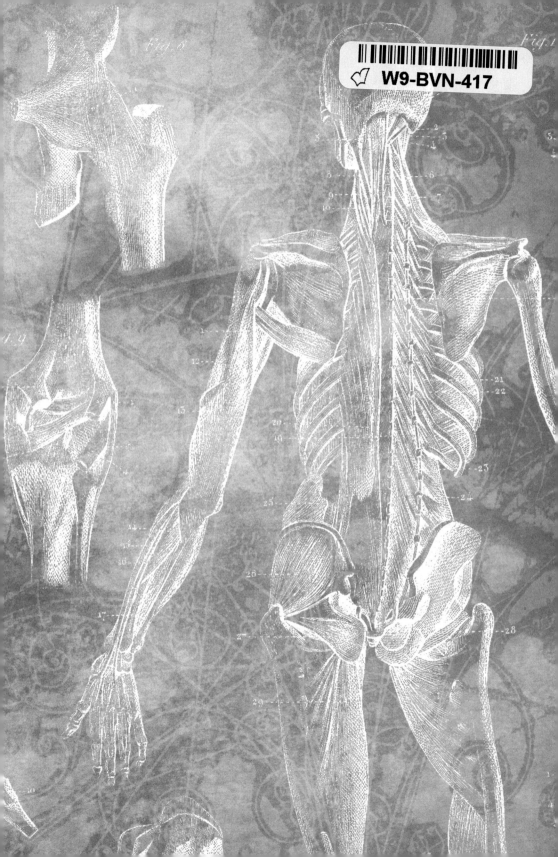

ON BEING HUMAN

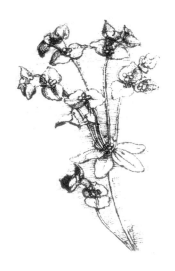

DAISAKU IKEDA

RENÉ SIMARD • GUY BOURGEAULT

ON BEING HUMAN

Where Ethics, Medicine and Spirituality Converge

MIDDLEWAY

P R E S S

Published by Middleway Press
A division of SGI-USA
606 Wilshire Boulevard, Santa Monica, CA 90401

Originally published in an English hardcover edition by Les Presses de l'Université de Montréal, 2002

Cover design by Dunn and Associates

10   9   8   7   6   5   4   3

Library of Congress Cataloging-in-Publication Data

Ikeda, Daisaku.
  On being human : where ethics, medicine, and spirituality converge on being human /
Daisaku Ikeda, René [i.e. Renâe] Simard, Guy Bourgeault.
      p. cm.
Originally published: Montreal : Les Presses de l'Université de
Montréal, 2002.
Includes index.
  ISBN 0-9723267-1-5 (Softcover)
  1. Health--Religious aspects--Buddhism. 2. Medical ethics--Religious aspects--Buddhism. 3.
Bioethics--Religious aspects--Buddhism. 4. Buddhism--Doctrines. I. Simard, René. II.
Bourgeault, Guy, 1933-
  BQ4570.M4I324 2003
  179.7--dc22
                                        2003014076

Table of Contents

Acknowledgements

The authors would like to thank everyone who helped bring about the discussions reflected in these pages and all those who contributed to this publication, especially Tadashi Ohira, Vice-President of SGI-Canada, who played the role of Montreal-Tokyo liaison and devoted himself tirelessly to supporting and facilitating our dialogue; Dr. Yoichi Kawada, Director of the Institute of Oriental Philosophy in Tokyo; translators Tsutomu Kano and Richard Gage; SGI interpreters Ryoko Yakura and Rie Tsumura who provided invaluable assistance at our meetings in Tokyo and Montreal; Helen Kandarakis, who translated some of the original French texts into English to ensure a smooth follow-through after our meetings in Tokyo; Jean Chapdelaine Gagnon, who skillfully translated and edited the French edition; the Ushio Publishing Company, under the direction of Kentaro Nishihara, which published our discussions in Japanese under the title *Kenko-to-Jinsei-Shoro-Byoshi-o-Kataru*; and the staff at Les Presses de l'Université de Montréal, who worked together to produce the hardcover edition of this book and to Middleway Press, who produced the paperback edition.

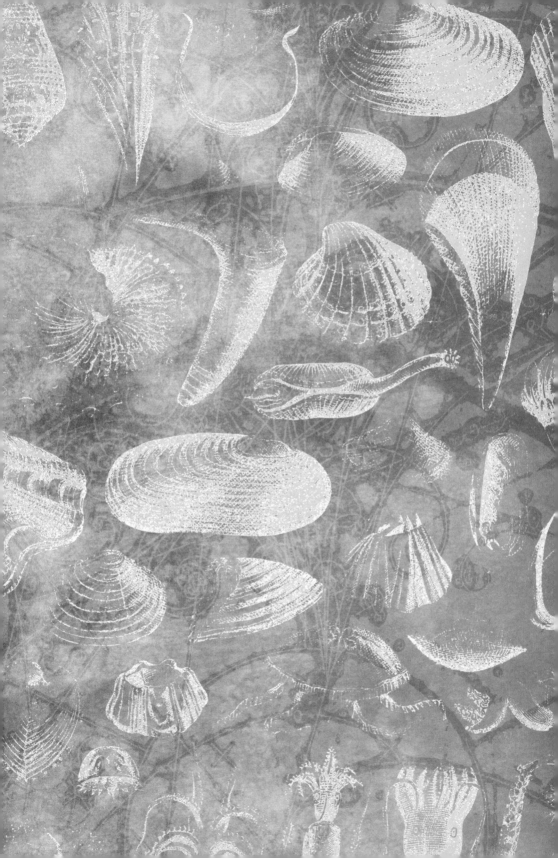

Preface

Each man's own life is the subject-matter of the art of living.
—Epictetus[1]

HEALTH is one of humankind's greatest preoccupations as we enter the twenty-first century, and I have often spoken of health in the light of Buddhist perspectives on life. In *On Being Human*, I am pleased to present the views of the eminent medical scientist René Simard, rector of the University of Montreal from 1993 to 1998, and the outstanding bioethicist Guy Bourgeault, professor of ethics at the same institution.

Rapid scientific and technological breakthroughs have enabled modern civilization to make great strides toward what could be termed "happiness." We have eradicated many of the ills that have long afflicted humankind, including numerous infectious diseases. Highly specialized techniques in other areas, particularly surgery, now enable us to heal pathological conditions once considered incurable.

The twenty-first century has been hailed as an age of biotechnology. Treatments for cancer, AIDS, cardiac disorders, and other intractable diseases will advance steadily, buoyed by the fruits of the latest medical technology designed for application to cells and genes and encroaching on the functions of the brain itself. Biotechnology has

1. *Epictetus: The Discourses as Reported by Arrian*, Book I, Chapter 15. Tr. W.A. Oldfather. Cambridge: Harvard University Press. 1925.

already opened up serious and wide-ranging medical ethics issues. We find ourselves facing questions dealing with brain death, dignified death, prenatal identification of genetic conditions associated with certain disorders, and in-vitro fertilization, to name only a few. Because of its effects on birth, aging, sickness and death, technology has entered the fundamental domain of life.

The ever-accelerating pace of social change imposes intense mental stress on us as human beings, sapping our inner spiritual strength and leading to depression and other mental disorders—including what could be called "sickness of the soul."

Spiritual torpor sets in as people separate themselves from nature—losing their place of refuge and retreat—and as physical aggression becomes more commonplace. Given the combination of negative and positive consequences of modern technological civilization, it is perhaps natural for people of our time to become increasingly concerned about health, one of the keys to happiness.

As a Buddhist, I have long pondered ways to promote the physical, mental, and spiritual well-being of the human race. My encounters with Dr. Simard and Dr. Bourgeault have provided an excellent opportunity to probe this question more deeply. Dr. Simard is a world-renowned authority on cancer, and Dr. Bourgeault is an expert not only on ethics and education, but also on Christian theology.

Relying on Dr. Simard's specialized knowledge of current research, we plunge immediately into a medical discussion of cancer and AIDS. But discrimination against the sick exacerbates the problem of illness, and human rights issues must be considered. Here, Dr. Bourgeault and I have much to contribute from the standpoint of ethics and the Buddhist view of life.

Next we consider the fundamental issue of nature and harmonious coexistence, moving on to deal with the specific issues of brain death, dignified death, and the ethical dilemmas of fertility and childbirth. Discussions of life itself—its origins, evolution, and the birth of humankind—and where we go from here bring us to the final chapter, "Dawn of the Century of Life." We ask the reader to envisage a century in which life is supreme. To bring humankind to such a century, how must we protect ourselves from the pathological character of modern society? What new conceptions of humanity, what new cosmologies can guide us in the new millennium?

All three of us hope that the twenty-first century will be a "Century of Life," a time when science and spirituality resonate together to create a sound, balanced, and wholesome civilization.

Finally, I hope that our thoughts here will arouse echoes in the reader's mind, serve as a rich source of material for reflection, and contribute to the building of a wholesome, humane civilization, where spirituality illumines every life.

DAISAKU IKEDA, *President*
SOKA GAKKAI INTERNATIONAL

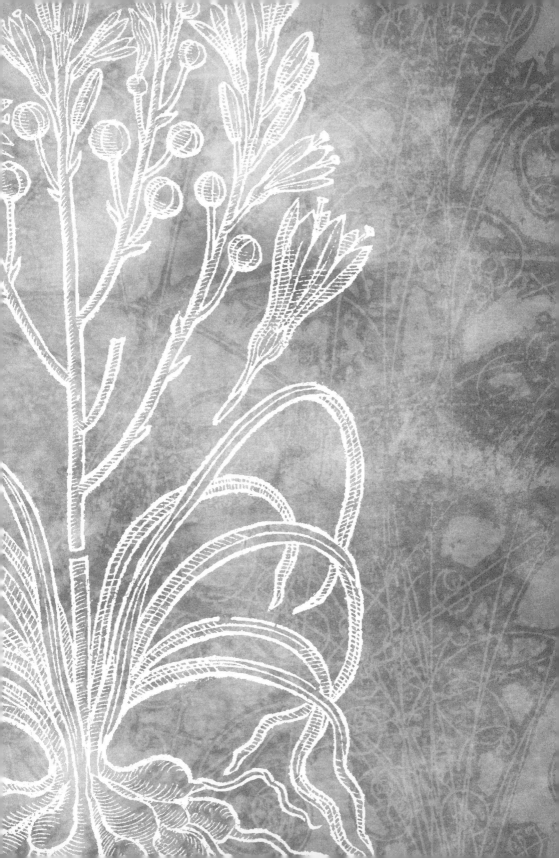

Foreword

M Y FIRST ENCOUNTER with President Ikeda was back in the spring of 1990: we met as part of an exchange between Soka University and the University of Montreal, on the occasion of the signing of a letter of agreement between the two institutions. The Soka Gakkai International of Canada had given me the opportunity to read a thoughtful book by President Ikeda entitled *Life: An Enigma, a Precious Jewel*, and I was struck by the author's bold and profound analysis of the origin of life and the diversity of species, and intrigued by the new dimension oriental philosophy offers to the laws of evolution.

When Mr. Ikeda and I met, we had a lengthy discussion on the effect that recent advances in molecular biology and genetics would have on accepted explanations for the origin of life and on the answers to such fundamental questions as, Where do we come from? Who are we? and Where are we going? We talked about the differences between harmony (normal growth and development) and chaos (malignant growth and cancer development). We agreed on the social responsibility of scientists and the importance of higher education. Mr. Ikeda, the founder of Soka University, and I compared the content and organization of educational programs, agreed on the value of student exchanges, and discussed the need to internationalize our institutions. Later, when I visited Soka University, its campus and facilities impressed me greatly.

We discovered that we have a great deal in common, even though our cultural and scientific backgrounds are different. Mr. Ikeda impressed me both as a human being who cares about people suffering from illness, stress, and environmental degradation, and as an open-minded philosopher steeped in culture. We came to the conclusion that an encounter between a philosopher and a biologist could produce an interesting dialogue. For one thing, biology is making many discoveries that carry us to ethical frontiers, and require enlightened social management. For another, philosophy is the root of all disciplines. The universities of the world recognize its supremacy by calling their most elevated degree that of doctor of philosophy—*Philosophiae Doctor*.

We also decided that input from an eminent scholar with top credentials in bioethics and education would add another appealing dimension to our dialogue. Therefore, we invited Professor Guy Bourgeault of the University of Montreal to join us. His contribution proved invaluable.

President Ikeda insisted that we avoid scientific jargon and use easily understandable language in our discussions. Certain scientific details are inevitable in a work of this kind, but the reader can rest assured that they are broached in entirely accessible terms.

This book deals with health, disease, bioethics, and education, focusing on the problems of cancer and AIDS. At last our work has come to fruition, in spite of distances separating the authors, language differences, and heavy workloads. The editor has lightened our task considerably. We are greatly indebted to him for his constant encouragement and attentiveness.

RENÉ SIMARD, *Rector*,
UNIVERSITY OF MONTREAL

Introduction

IKEDA • Dr. René Simard, who was until recently rector of the University of Montreal, has become a world authority in the field of physiology and cytobiology for his research on cancer and in particular as a pioneer in research on antimetabolites and anticancer agents. Dr. Bourgeault is a professor of bioethics and pedagogy. Their respective fields of research will be areas of vital concern in the twenty-first century. They have kindly agreed to share with us their knowledge and experience to help deepen our understanding of the four universal sufferings of birth, old age, sickness, and death, and to learn how to lead a healthy life.

SIMARD • I feel this dialogue is a valuable opportunity to encourage cancer and AIDS sufferers and people concerned about the impact of technological breakthroughs on their own lives. I have had many chances to meet and exchange views with you, Mr. Ikeda, and I must say I have found our discussions very stimulating.

IKEDA • The University of Montreal and Soka University began an academic and educational exchange program in 1994. Since then, to my great pleasure as founder of Soka University, the relationship between the two institutions has become closer and deeper.

In April 1994, the *Centre d'études de l'Asie de l'Est* (Center for East

Asian Studies) at your university and the Institute of Oriental Philosophy, of which I am founder, concluded a scholarly exchange agreement. Dr. Simard, you honored us by attending and speaking at the signing ceremony. On that occasion, you said, "Harmony between truth and science is a real contribution to humanity." These words aptly express the spirit and meaning of our dialogue.

BOURGEAULT · Relations between Canada and Japan were gravely affected by the 1939–45 war, when our countries were ranked as enemies. Fortunately things have changed. I am very pleased that the exchange program between Soka University and the University of Montreal can bear witness to this, especially since our discussions will be part of the framework.

SIMARD · I will never forget my first visit to Soka University in 1990. A female student choir welcomed me with song. By now they must have all graduated, but I still have a vivid memory of that day.

That visit gave me a glimpse of your great achievements. The entire Soka campus breathes an atmosphere of openness to the world, infectious goodwill and harmony. I could see that the university instills more than knowledge: it produces fully rounded individuals. And what a wonderful cultural environment it lavishes on the students, who always have access to such resources as the splendid Tokyo Fuji Art Museum and its superb collection!

IKEDA · Thank you for your kind words. But the University of Montreal, too, is a world-class institution.

SIMARD · With 50,000 students and 13 faculties, including the graduate school, it is the largest French-speaking university in America.

One of our university's distinctive features is the effort we devote to educational exchange. With global economic movements exerting such decisive influences, universities, too, are called upon to respond to the need for internationalism and diversification in both research and teaching. We are doing our best to answer that call. We have already concluded international student-exchange agreements with more than 90 institutions worldwide, including, of course, Soka University.

IKEDA · I also cherish the memory of my visit to your university during the fall of 1993. Soka Gakkai International (SGI) was launching its first overseas exhibit, "Toward a Century of Humanity: An Overview of Human Rights in Today's World," and I attended the opening ceremony. You were both a great help in making the exhibition possible.

SIMARD • It was our pleasure to provide space for that superb exhibition, which caused a great stir on campus. Human rights are one of the most important issues in the Western world today, and the SGI movement aims to protect human rights. No one should be allowed to deprive others of their rights.

IKEDA • The SGI human-rights exhibit has been held in 24 cities in eight countries so far and has been well received everywhere.

BOURGEAULT • The wide range of SGI activities—often devoted to studying solutions to crucial problems—is very impressive. You and your colleagues are clearly motivated by a strong sense of mission, and you seem to fear neither discussion nor action.

IKEDA • In *Choose Life*,[1] my dialogue with Arnold J. Toynbee (1889–1975), he said that the twentieth century would be remembered not as a period of political dissent or an era of technological breakthroughs, but as an epoch when the human community began considering the good health of all its members as a feasible objective.

Today societies are seriously preoccupied with health. This may be partly because peace is becoming a reality for more and more people. On the other hand, increasing levels of stress may contribute to a real rise in personal anxiety about health. In such an atmosphere, health has become a prime topic of debate and discussion. Some enterprising parties, relying on manifestly unscientific theories, are even exploiting the commercial possibilities of the health boom.

It seems to me that we need to set a course toward a clear conception of health, established not on self-interest but on valid philosophic and scientific bases, and then to spread that view widely in a manner that is easy for everyone to understand.

BOURGEAULT • Questions about life and death are of crucial importance. I am always surprised that bioethicists in North America and

1. *The Toynbee-Ikeda Dialogue: Choose Life.* London: Oxford University Press. 1976.

Europe seem to try to skirt them and deal only with more specific issues and technical matters.

IKEDA • To make the twenty-first century a "century of health," lay persons must become better advised and better informed. I am ready to do whatever I can to make that happen. The general public rarely reads essays and monographs. That is why I prefer to broach serious issues through dialogue, and why I have suggested the dialogue form for our exchange, because it makes ideas clear and accessible. Dialogue was the medium of Socrates (469–399 BCE). Both Shakyamuni[2] and Nichiren[3] (1222–82), whose teachings I follow, taught through dialogue. Drawing on that tradition, I have conducted dialogues on contemporary themes with many outstanding and influential people.

BOURGEAULT • At the beginning of your essay on brain death,[4] you expressed the wish that a better-informed public would participate in the health debate, which concerns everyone. The questions we are going to discuss—questions of life and health, illness and death—surely interest all human beings. I think that the dialogue form that you suggest is the perfect vehicle for discussions of such general interest.

IKEDA • I also hope our discussions will highlight the concerns of women. In the twenty-first century, women will undoubtedly move to the forefront. I sincerely hope that female readers will find our discussions relevant and interesting.

BOURGEAULT • You bring up a delicate subject that is all the more pertinent since our discussion will be among three men, without feminine participation. Regrettably, big issues are often debated solely among men. Without falling back on simplistic stereotypes, I think it can be said that men's ideas are often based on the notion of power understood and experienced as domination and control. Women are perhaps, in general, less obsessed by the play of economic and

---

2. Founder of Buddhism, the historic Buddha.

3. Founder of Nichiren Buddhism, the Buddha of the Latter Day of the Law.

4. Daisaku Ikeda. *Thoughts on the Problem of Death from the Viewpoint of the Buddhism of Nichiren Daishonin.* Tokyo: The Institute of Oriental Philosophy.

political interests. They are more open to analysis and to actions that are not directly dictated by power play. They seem to think more in terms of assisting life and improving its quality.

IKEDA • This is an idea that merits serious attention. For years, you have studied ways of drawing on "woman power" to improve the quality of human life. You have suggested that feminine power is rooted more in sharing, dialogue, and understanding than in control. I share your confidence in its potential, which you so aptly expressed when you said that we expect a great deal from the women's movement, not only for women, but for men too.

SIMARD • Many of the students who complete their studies at our medical school are women. A higher percentage of women complete their courses and receive their diplomas. And a higher percentage of these women than of their male classmates take on difficult and demanding jobs. The number of female physicians is rapidly increasing. In Canada, if current trends continue, 65% of medical doctors will soon be women. Women doctors are better communicators than their male counterparts. With an increase in their numbers, I think the patient-doctor relationship will improve.

IKEDA • We shall return to this important point. But to get the discussion started, I would first like to ask each of you some personal questions. Dr. Simard, please tell us a little about your childhood.

SIMARD • I was born and grew up in Montreal, Canada, the youngest child in a large family. Both my parents believed deeply in the importance of education and made sure that we all went to college and university. From my earliest youth, I was lucky enough to live in a rich cultural environment steeped in the humanistic traditions of Greek and Latin studies.

IKEDA • While you were studying at the University of Montreal, you switched from literature to medical science and received a doctoral degree in medicine. In the following years, you made a brilliant career in pathology, cytobiology, and oncology. What prompted you to go into these particular areas?

SIMARD • Originally, intense compassion for the sick led me to want to attend the medical faculty. But medical explanations

of the causes of illnesses left me unsatisfied, so I chose pathology as my area of specialization, because pathologists are the
ones who propose diagnoses as illnesses progress.

While there is no doubt that diagnoses are crucial, I soon realized that
the only criteria for the pathologists' all-important judgments are their
knowledge of biomorphology and accumulated data from past experience. Pathologists, however, rarely discuss the causes of illnesses. Therefore I ultimately chose to strike out into two areas that, just then, were
fields of active and promising research—cytobiology and genetics.

IKEDA • I see. And after completing studies at the University of Montreal,
you went on to do research in New York and Paris.

SIMARD • I left Canada in 1962, when I was 27, and went to New York
City to serve an internship at Mt. Sinai Hospital and Medical School,
which had a reputation as one of the best physician-training hospitals
in the United States. With the late Dr. Hans Popper (1903–88) as its
guiding light, the department of pathology was famous for the very
high quality and vitality of its research. I was fortunate to be able to
complete my training in pathology while working on a research
project on cell-division control.

For someone like me, eager to immerse myself in a new and progressive culture, New York City was the perfect environment. I remember
how much I was changed by simply being in the city.

Even now, New York has lost none of its lustre in my eyes.

IKEDA • You speak of it in almost poetic tones. And what about Paris?

SIMARD • I went to Paris three years later, in 1965, to take a research
position under Dr. Wilhelm Bernhard (1920–78).

Bernhard was a top-ranking scientist, very well known at the time.
He was famous for his work on cancer and was one of the first biologists to describe the retrovirus now known to cause AIDS. He was also
a philosopher with a wealth of experience; he could find meaning in
everyday life.

In 1965, Jacques Monod (1910–76), François Jacob (1920–), and
André Lwoff (1901–94) had just received the Nobel Prize in physiology, and Paris was a Mecca of cytobiological research. I had the good
fortune to be able to attend lectures by these giants and to meet them
personally on numerous occasions.

IKEDA • Monod's *Chance and Necessity*[5] was translated into Japanese and had considerable impact in Japan. I, too, found it extremely interesting.

Now, please tell us about the University of Montreal, of which you were rector. How would you describe its basic philosophy? What makes it unique?

SIMARD • The Latin motto of the University of Montreal is *"Fide splendet et scientia"* (May it shine with truth and knowledge). What could be more stimulating to a scientist than such a motto? Early in the 1990s, the university issued an official document clarifying its mission, and the top priorities are described as pioneering in new areas of knowledge and meeting rigid standards of training for students working toward master's degrees and doctorates.

Our faculty members are required to dedicate themselves wholeheartedly to research in their fields, to remain in the vanguard of scholarship, and to incorporate the results of their work into their courses. Every year, the university confers 300 doctorates, and more than 2,000 candidates receive master's degrees. In addition to 13 faculties and 2 affiliated institutions, the university has about 120 chairs in diverse fields, research centers, and interdisciplinary research groups.

About c$200 million is allocated to the university for research every year. In this way, our university makes an important contribution to the economic development of Montreal, Quebec, and Canada. About one-quarter of the available funds is used for contract research for private corporations and joint ventures.

It was an extraordinary privilege to serve as rector of the University of Montreal. I sincerely believe that as rector I was invested with the mission of making our university "shine with truth and knowledge." During my term in office, my sole objective was to work toward fulfilling that ideal.

IKEDA • To change the subject slightly, I'd like to ask you whom you hold in highest esteem.

SIMARD • I have had the great good fortune to associate with and get to know a number of world-famous professors and scientists whose lives are truly worthy of admiration. If I have to choose only one, it

---

5. Jacques Monod. *Chance and Necessity: An Essay on the Natural Philosophy of Modern Biology.* New York: Vintage. 1971.

would have to be Dr. Wilhelm Bernhard.

IKEDA • He was your mentor in Paris? You just pointed out that he was one of the first biologists to describe the retrovirus now known to cause AIDS and leukemia.

SIMARD • That is correct. I received rigorous training in scientific methodology in his laboratory, where I also conducted my initial research on the structure and function of cell nuclei (cytoblasts).

Dr. Bernhard was a very ardent man. His enthusiasm for research, the arts, plants, and people was extraordinary. He maintained a passion for all these things simultaneously, and rather than keeping his enthusiasm to himself, he communicated it widely in passionate speeches and fervent discussions. People around him found themselves infected by his contagious enthusiasm almost before they realized what was happening. His tone of voice, the keenness in his eyes— everything about him was electrifying and inspiring.

IKEDA • In Buddhism, an encounter with a mentor, a person whose ideals one shares and inherits, is considered the surest route to genuine happiness. Dr. Simard, you are very fortunate to have encountered such an extraordinary person.

SIMARD • Dr. Bernhard was not just an outstanding scientist, but also a humanist with a genuine and very obvious love for other people, for humanity. He was highly cultivated, a man with universal interests and penetrating knowledge, and throughout his whole life he waged the meaningful battle of the true world citizen. Looking back over his life, he wrote: "I was born Swiss at a linguistic frontier. For many years I have lived as a Frenchman deeply rooted in Paris. I think as a European, and I dream as a citizen of the world."

IKEDA • To dream as a citizen of the world—that is precisely what my mentor Josei Toda (1900–58) taught his students when he introduced them to his global-family concept. He urged young people to build a global human community and live as world citizens. I have dedicated my life to the realization of my mentor's vision.

SIMARD • In Bernhard's laboratory, I learned how much he appreciated encounters and interactions with other people. For over 30 years, he happily passed on his knowledge to young research students and colleagues who came from all over the world to learn from him. He considered sharing knowledge with others as important as acquiring new knowledge for himself. In that sense, he showed himself to be as great an educator as a scientist.

IKEDA • Dr. Bernhard's spirit of service embodies the Buddhist ideal of compassion. Truly great people dedicate their whole lives to the love of their fellow human beings—to the unlimited love of humanity—regardless of their personal circumstances or sufferings.

Mahatma Gandhi (1869–1948) and Rabindranath Tagore (1861–1941) were such men, and I would venture to include Tsunesaburo Makiguchi (1871–1944), the founding president of Soka Gakkai, and Josei Toda, second president, among those who gave their lives for the love of humankind.

People of noble character, like your mentor, Dr. Bernhard, are sound in body, mind and soul; they radiate the humanistic spirit. The Buddhist term *bodhisattva* indicates people of noble character who devote themselves to helping others. People with the bodhisattva nature probably suffer neither anxiety nor fear at death, the ultimate suffering, because their lives are filled with the joy and satisfaction of having lived for the well-being of others.

SIMARD • That is certainly true. For his epitaph, Bernhard chose the following words of the French philosopher and historian Ernest Renan (1823–92). They beautifully sum up Bernhard's own thought. "Only the end deserves consideration: all else is vanity. He has lived most who has loved most in spirit, heart, and deeds."[6]

IKEDA • A profound truth. Nichiren Daishonin taught us: "First learn about death, and then about other matters."[7] According to one saying, people die as they have lived. Be that as it may, a person's whole life is revealed at the moment of the final reckoning. The Buddhist teaching that the quality or condition of life persists even after death only emphasizes the importance of life's final chapter.

People who love with the most all-consuming fervor are those who live life to the fullest, regardless of how long their physical existence lasts. To invest one's heart and soul in caring for others, to burn with

6. Ernest Renan. *L'avenir de la science.* Paris: Lévy ed. 1890. Free translation.
7. *Gosho Zenshu.* Tokyo: Soka Gakkai. 1952. 1404.

passionate love for humanity, that is what Buddhists call the "bodhisattva way." I believe this kind of perfect life constitutes the way to optimum health and true longevity.

Let me now ask Dr. Bourgeault some personal questions. I believe you, too, were born in Montreal?

BOURGEAULT • Yes, and I have spent most of my life in an urban environment. I am a city boy at heart. I love the sea, lakes, rivers, fields, and forests—I can spend hours gazing at the sea, calm or rough, or listening to the wind in the trees—but after that, I must return to the bustle of the city and its busy crowds. I delight in the streets of Montreal and even more so in those of Rome, Paris and, recently, Tokyo.

I am a literary person. I studied philosophy and theology. My research and teaching have dealt with ethics, especially bioethics and education. Still I remain a literary person. I often find my ethical and educational points of reference in the Bible, the great tragedies of Greek antiquity, and more recent French literature. Literary works take into consideration the complexity, ambiguity, and contradiction of reality—things the scientific viewpoint, which dissects reality, often overlooks.

IKEDA • Fictional literature—including poetry—is born of an intuitive perception of reality as a whole, which literature depicts as it unfolds. Science, on the other hand, analyzes reality, seeking to identify its parts or elements and understand the relationships among them. Literature, poetry, philosophy, religion, and science are all invaluable spiritual assets, but I find poetry and other forms of literature most compelling.

BOURGEAULT • I have read some of your books and poems—in French or English translation, unfortunately, not in Japanese. A common theme seems to be present in all of them: the importance of sharing and our common membership in a nature that exceeds us.

IKEDA • Nothing exists in isolation, neither in nature nor in the world of humans. All things are related and dependent on each other. Together they form the prodigious cosmos. Good literature, prose or poetry, connects us humans with nature and the cosmos, integrating us into them in a way that can heal our souls when reality weighs on them or tears at them. The poetic spirit, I believe, enables us to perceive our own presence in the universal vastness, where everything is unified.

After your university studies, you became a priest in the Catholic Church. Then, twenty years later, you left the priesthood to pursue research in ethics, particularly bioethics.

BOURGEAULT · The same things that led me into the priesthood later led me elsewhere: a mixture of liberty, sometimes nonconformity, and a commitment with—rather than to—others. Probably I am indebted to my modest origins and my personal rootedness for my interest in social questions and in what is called social justice and the defense of rights and freedoms. Professionally, I try first of all to focus on the social and political dimensions of ethical and educational issues.

My career has developed along the lines of education and ethics. I believe that fundamentally education is ethical work and ethics is a work of education—of ourselves, not of others. We cannot educate others: we educate ourselves with others . . .

IKEDA · You have just put your finger on a vital issue in education today. In an essay on improving the quality of life, you asked a question that is critical for all of us: "How should human beings live?"

BOURGEAULT · Life is the pleasure of living. It is tension, a forward march toward something we cannot exactly identify because the horizon is always receding. There is no meaning to life but life itself, no other goal but life itself—with all its difficulties and absurdities and the despair they sometimes bring, and with its solidarities that constitute the fabric and the prize of our thread of encounters, exchanges, and battles.

IKEDA · I think I'm beginning to understand your basic outlook on life.

BOURGEAULT · The momentum of life is sometimes thwarted. The absurd horrors the news bombards us with day after day—wars, catastrophes, rapes, and carnage—are unbearable. I long cherished the ideal, despite all indications to the contrary, that the human conscience grows more refined as liberty, equality, and fraternity progress. But I have been obliged to kiss that particular delusion goodbye. I have had to accept that history can be—and is—written in facts, with no obligatory advance from worse to better—or even to less bad—and with no set direction other than the one given by the person who lives, breathes, and hopes in spite of all reasons to despair. I love the obstinacy of the living.

IKEDA • Your words make a noble idea almost tangible.

Now, I would like to ask you the same question that I asked Dr. Simard earlier: Who has influenced you most in your life?

BOURGEAULT • Two of my college professors made great impressions on me. One was Julien Laperrière, who taught me literature—poetry and the novel. Later, when I had become a teacher myself, I met him again in a setting in which we could discuss the theater. I still remember a poem he read aloud to us one day, beautifully and passionately. It was a poem that he especially loved and we were supposed to analyze it, but he stopped us, fearing our analysis would destroy the poem's life and beauty.

IKEDA • What a wonderfully revealing anecdote! Perhaps your professor wanted you to fully experience the essential differences between poetry and science. Like Dr. Simard, you were very fortunate to discover such an exceptional mentor. Few things are as extraordinary as encountering a unique being who inspires in us the desire to emulate.

BOURGEAULT • Claude Labelle, another of my professors, also made a strong impression, perhaps less for what he actually taught us than for the attention he gave to what we were thinking and doing and for his desire to push us to go farther. No doubt part of my conception of education comes from him.

IKEDA • Shakyamuni said that only a few are ever privileged to encounter a great teacher; those who never do are numerous beyond counting. He goes on to say, "Only a few listen to what a teacher imparts; many pay no attention to the teaching." This is very true. Encountering a great teacher does not guarantee learning. It is necessary to listen, assimilate the master's teachings and then put them into practice. Students should demonstrate gratitude to their teacher by their eagerness to respond and to act in accordance with the teachings.

Dr. Bourgeault, you encountered two great teachers in your youth and today you practice what you learned from them.

BOURGEAULT • But I learned not only from professors of literature. I am also greatly indebted to, for example, Léo Cormier (1924–84), a highly committed social worker whom I met when he was president of the Quebec League of Rights and Liberties. From him—or with him—I learned the importance of an idea that nourishes itself on action, which in turn it directs. In my life I have learned—and am still learning—from many people, students and friends alike.

IKEDA • Besides your two cherished teachers, you had good friends. Wisdom gained and enriched in the context of daily life—that is just what is meant by the "wisdom of people." Subtle powers of observation honed by adversity and the need to cope with real problems make it possible to see the essence of things. This is authentic wisdom. Recognizing and respecting differences and learning the quality of the other are the marks of true friendship.

BOURGEAULT • I am glad that this dialogue will give me a chance to get to know your opinions on several important issues and to understand better what our epoch can draw from Buddhist traditions.

IKEDA • According to Buddhist thought, "Life as a unity of body and spirit goes on eternally (*shikishin-renji*)."[8] When spirit and body work together in harmony, life continues moving toward fulfilment, realizing itself more fully at each upward turn. This is the ideal of human life. Of course, physical health is important, but so are mental and spiritual health, not to mention the health of society.

In this series of discussions, we will ask ourselves many questions. What is a truly meaningful life? How can we lead a healthy life, which is a necessary condition for happiness? What can medical science tell us about the fulfilled life? What can we learn from Buddhist wisdom? I hope that our answers to these and other questions result in a lively discussion that captures the interest of the people of the twenty-first century.

---

8. *Life as a psychosomatic entity continues eternally:* The great Chinese scholar T'ien-t'ai, famous for his commentaries on the Lotus Sutra, uses this expression in the last chapter of the fourth volume of his *Words and Phrases of the Lotus Sutra* to explain the impurity of life. The expression describes an important aspect of Buddhist thought that posits that people maintain, lifetime after lifetime, the changing and uncertain form of their bodies and spirits.

CHAPTER ONE

CANCER AND AIDS

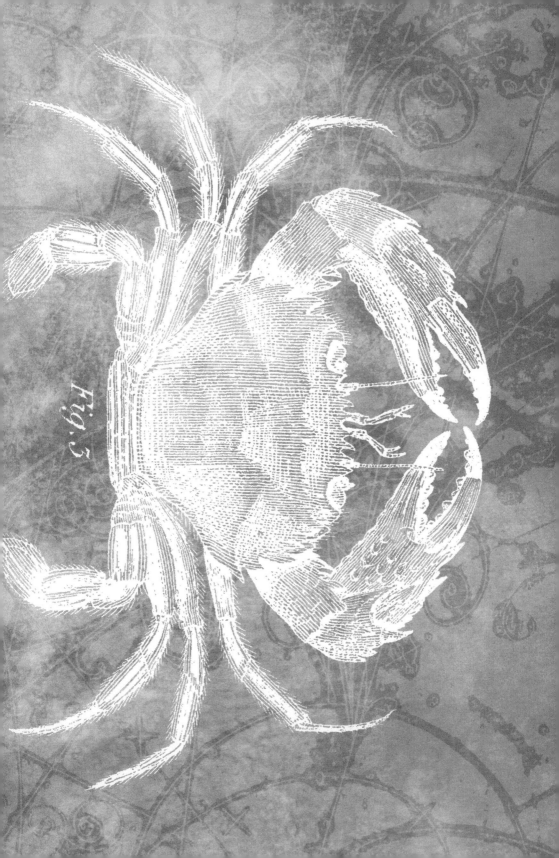

Fig. 5

1. Cancer Past and Present

Hippocrates and liberation from divine fiat

IKEDA • Cancer and AIDS are undoubtedly the illnesses that cause the most concern these days, as they continue to stymie treatments and medical research alike. At the same time, cloning is seen as a harbinger of promising progress by some, and as a great danger by others. I thought we could begin our discussions by speaking of cancer, AIDS and cloning.

Dr. Simard, as a world-renowned specialist in cancer research, you surely agree that one of the dearest wishes of humankind is a cure for cancer. I once participated in a discussion on the life of Napoleon Bonaparte (1769–1821) with a group of French historians, and we debated the theory that he died of stomach cancer.

SIMARD • Yes, that is what some experts say. Researching the distant past, scientists have found traces of cancer as far back as the Egyptian mummies. We tend to think of cancer as a modern disease, but it seems to have come into the world at the same time as the emergence of our species. It was definitely present in ancient, even prehistoric, times.

IKEDA • I suppose there must be all kinds of evidence and documentation on the subject. Do you know when human beings first recognized the existence of cancer?

SIMARD • The ancient Greeks at the time of the great physician Hippocrates (ca. 460–ca. 375 BCE) had already identified it. Hippocrates referred to cancer as *karkinos*, or crab, from which we get our word *carcinoma* for malignant tumors. Ignorant of the cause of cancer, the Greeks aptly imagined it as an evil crab burrowing deeper and deeper into its victim, devouring the flesh along its way until nothing was left to consume.

IKEDA • Since medical scientists today are still searching for the causes of cancer, it is not surprising that the ancient Greeks did not know how or why cancers grew. Even so, they left very precise descriptions of its symptoms and the course of its progress.

SIMARD • Before the time of Hippocrates, human destiny was believed to be in the hands of the gods. Since disease, too, was believed to be destined by fate, the best people could do was to try to find out—through oracles, mediums, fortune-tellers, and the like—what fate held in store for them. Sometimes people offered sacrifices to deities to appease their anger.

IKEDA • At about the same time as Hippocrates, in India, too, religious rites assumed great importance. At the peak of its authoritarianism and corruption, the priestly Brahman caste threatened the ordinary people with hell for refusing to perform certain religious rites. Apparently, conditions were similar in the East and the West in the fifth century BCE.

Shakyamuni began a religious movement to liberate people from the corrupt clergy. Jivaka, one of Shakyamuni's followers and a physician comparable to Hippocrates, laid the foundations for the Buddhist art of healing.

SIMARD • In Hellenic Greece, Hippocrates was the first to establish a clear distinction between medicine and prayer. He theorized that disease was a natural rather than supernatural phenomenon, unrelated to religion or magic. He applied all his knowledge and experience to objectively defining symptoms of illnesses and explaining them in terms of the well-known notion of the four bodily humors—blood, phlegm, black bile, and choler (yellow bile). He claimed that black bile, thought to be produced by the spleen and the stomach, was the etiologic agent of cancer.

Hippocrates set medicine on its proper course by distancing it from mystical healing and orienting it toward the formation of a diagnostic method centered on observation and comparison of symptoms, analysis of causes, and—on the bases of these—prognosis of a disease's progression.

IKEDA • Speaking of Hippocrates, in my discussions with Arnold Toynbee, he strongly suggested that people training for any profession, not just medicine, should take a kind of Hippocratic Oath.

SIMARD • As you know, everyone training to be a physician must take the Hippocratic Oath before being officially recognized as a medical doctor. Considering how much all humanity owes to Hippocrates, this is not surprising. Taking the meaning of the oath to heart, new doctors learn to respect patients and recognize the importance of clinical observation. They become aware of the absolute necessity of reflecting on the ethical aspects of the medical profession.

IKEDA • That makes very good sense. The ethical dimension is extremely important.

Age and geography as factors in the incidence of cancer

IKEDA • As people live longer, the incidence of cancer naturally increases correspondingly. Do you think that—apart from higher numbers due to increasing longevity—we will see overall cancer rates climb even higher?

SIMARD • Well, as you say, the incidence of cancer rises as a population ages. Statistics on rates of sickness and death from cancer must be adjusted to reflect this reality.

Nonetheless, if we are to trust the statistics—available back to the 1930s—and make adjustments in the numerical values for certain types of cancer, the mortality rate seems not to have changed appreciably. Lung cancer is the big exception. In its case, the mortality rate has risen considerably in the last forty years.

IKEDA • How many types of cancer are known so far? Are there regional differences in the incidence of cancer?

SIMARD • There are about 250 types of cancer, all with differing incidences. Some types are known to be more prevalent in certain regions or among certain age groups.

Cancer of the liver, for example, occurs with greater frequency in Africa and Southeast Asia than elsewhere. Among industrialized countries, Japan is the only one with a high rate of stomach cancer. Elsewhere, this kind of cancer is decreasing. Cancer of the esophagus is comparatively widespread in South China, Iran, and Normandy. Developing countries generally have fairly high rates of cervical cancer; but, as if it were an economic indicator, the rate begins to drop as soon as development picks up. Among Australians of British extraction melanoma is much more common than in other populations. On the other hand, the incidence of prostate cancer is linked to age.

IKEDA · In Japan, stomach cancer is still the most prevalent type, although deaths from it are on the decline. Liver and pancreatic cancers are also frequent. All told, cancer of the digestive system accounts for 70% of the total. Breast cancer, too, has been rising rapidly in recent years.

SIMARD · Statistics show no less than 125,000 new cancer cases diagnosed in Canada in 1995 and more than 60,000 cancer-related deaths. More than half the newly diagnosed cases fell into three categories. In women, the most common types were breast cancer, lung cancer, and colorectal cancer. In men, prostate cancer, lung cancer, rectal cancer and colon cancer. Breast cancer remained the most frequently diagnosed cancer among women, and prostate cancer among men. Lung cancer, however, was once again the principal cause of death.

The probabilities of contracting or dying of cancer in Canada are as follows. For women, breast cancer will strike one in nine, rectal or colon cancer one in sixteen, and lung cancer one in twenty-two. Prostate cancer will strike more than one man in ten—especially men over seventy. One man in eleven will suffer from lung cancer.

Cancer in children and adults

IKEDA · In Japan, only accidents kill more children than cancer does. The most common cancer among children is leukemia. Juvenile cancer is the source of intense suffering for the stricken children themselves and unfathomable anguish for parents and families.

SIMARD · Thirty years ago, a diagnosis of juvenile leukemia was received as almost a death sentence. The child was usually expected to die in less than two years. Today half of children with cancer or leukemia recover completely. The frequency of recovery varies with the type of the disease. Even when cures are incomplete, a great many children can hope to live longer thanks to continuous treatments that combat and reduce symptoms.

The process is long and slow, but a perceptible increase in successful treatments can be discerned in the growing number of children who are, sooner or later, completely cured by therapy. Nothing can give greater pleasure to pediatricians, parents, families, and nurses who have seen so many young lives sacrificed on the altar of cancer and who, at each death, have felt as if a part of themselves died as well.

IKEDA • Is there a difference between the cancer that strikes children and the cancer that develops in adults?

SIMARD • Most of the recent medical breakthroughs in the study and treatment of cancer concern the illness in children and young adults. Since the end of the 1960s, the number of total remissions has steadily increased. This success has encouraged further research, giving all children and young people who suffer from cancer new reasons to hope.

I think we can conclude, on a relatively conjectural basis, that juvenile and adult cancers are generally not the same disease. The types of cancer diagnosed in children usually are infrequent tumors accompanied by scattered symptoms. In almost all cases of complete remission, total cure comes within two years after the first manifestation of the illness. When cancer strikes an adult, on the other hand, the sickness does not progress particularly fast. As a general rule, no long-term–survival prognosis for an adult cancer patient can be made with certainty until five years after diagnosis.

Both death and remission occur more quickly in juvenile and early-adulthood cancer than in patients of advanced age. In fact, the characteristics of cancer in children and young adults are closely related to the classic characteristics of contagious sicknesses observed since the time of Louis Pasteur (1822–95).

Oncogenes in normal cells

IKEDA • Tell me candidly, in the twenty-first century, will cancer cease being the disease that universally evokes the fear of death?

SIMARD • In all parts of the world, cancer has become the second most common cause of death, after cardiovascular disease. Many of the contagious and endemic diseases of the past have been virtually eradicated from the face of the Earth. But cancer has taken their place, rapidly acquiring a fearsome reputation and becoming a formidable foe. Unfortunately, the battle to overcome it promises to be long.

IKEDA • The presence of carcinogens and oncogenes in the cells is thought to be one cause of cancer. How much do scientists understand about the process that transforms normal cells into cancerous cells?

SIMARD • We still have a long way to go before we can explain the mechanism that initially induces cancer in a healthy cell. For example, about twenty-five years ago chemical substances—carcinogens—were thought to cause cancer.

IKEDA • I believe your mentor, Dr. Bernhard, energetically advocated the theory of viral carcinogenesis.

SIMARD • Yes, that is right. Soon after people began looking into carcinogens, interest in the theory of viral carcinogenesis increased. Some researchers showed that certain viral genes cause cancer. They called them oncogenes. Later normal human cells were discovered to contain genes identical to these viral genes. To distinguish them from viral oncogenes, they were called proto-oncogenes.

IKEDA • The discovery of proto-oncogenes in normal human cells was big news.

SIMARD • It really was. But we still do not know what activates oncogenes or how they are controlled. The prevailing assumption is that other genes (anti-oncogenes) control oncogenes and suppress the onset of the abnormal cell proliferation we call cancer. But the details of the mechanism at play escape us.

Interestingly, scientists have now begun returning to chemical substances—carcinogens—in their search for the causes of cancer. In other words, theories about how cancer arises have come full circle without yet leading to any definitive answers. Perhaps the sphinx of cancer has not yet met her Oedipus, but sooner or later the day will come. What we will be in a position to do once we possess the secret is another story.

IKEDA • I suppose the confusion of the current state of affairs makes forecasts impossible.

SIMARD • Exactly. That is why my first lecture of each semester is always called "Harmony and Chaos." Normally, nine months after conception, a human life comes into the world endowed with an enormous range of possibilities. As the individual person grows, however, the harmonious condition of the cells can be transformed into a state of chaos. Such chaotic cells are thought to have the potential for carcinogenesis.

IKEDA • This idea contains deep insight into the essence of life itself. Buddhists emphasize harmony as the healthy life state. When it resonates in dynamic harmony, life radiates creativity.

Like ancient Greek, Indian, and Chinese healing arts, Buddhist medicine teaches that the body is composed of four elements: earth, fire, water, and wind. When the four are provisionally brought together in dynamic harmony, there is life. Various sicknesses occur when the harmony is disrupted. Death ensues when the harmony is irrevocably broken.

Though Buddhist and Western medical systems differ, they both interpret life phenomena in terms of harmony and dissonance.

2. Prevention and Treatment

The two most important factors:
Poor diet and smoking

IKEDA • We are told that the recovery rate from many types of cancer rises sharply when the disease is detected at an early stage. What methods are used nowadays to detect and diagnose cancer? Generally the very mention of medical examinations gives people pause. A clear understanding of the nature and purpose of the examinations, however, might make them less hesitant.

SIMARD • Prevention is divided into primary and secondary modes. Early detection and diagnosis are part of secondary prevention.

The aim of primary prevention is to eliminate causative factors or circumstances before the disease actually develops. Since some factors that lead to cancer are already well known, primary prevention focuses on trying to neutralize these factors and avoid creating or stimulating conditions in which cancer is likely to occur.

In order of importance, these factors are carcinogens (including cigarettes and cigars); industrial chemicals; ultraviolet rays and in rare cases radiation and x-rays; papilloma, herpes, and AIDS viruses; such infectious viruses as Epstein-Barr (EB) virus; diet; and heredity.

IKEDA • In Japan, the relationship between smoking and cancer is most frequently cited.

SIMARD • Today we thoroughly understand the causal connection between smoking and cancer, and smoking and cardiovascular disease. I would say that almost all citizens in the industrialized world are aware of the connection by now. The trouble is that, while perfectly aware of the risk they are taking, many people either choose to continue smoking or are too dependent to break the habit. We have been simply unable to intervene effectively. More and more young people are smoking, particularly adolescents and young women.

People in less developed countries lack ready access to reports, information, or articles about life style. It is hard to know to what extent they are informed—if at all—about the dangers of smoking.

Concrete information is now available to help formulate preventative measures against skin cancer resulting from overexposure to the sun. The frequency of skin cancer is growing, and we are seeing more cases of highly malignant melanoma. A large number of cases of less serious skin cancer, too, are being cited. So far, the best primary prevention for these types of cancer is education that presents convincing evidence and easy-to-understand explanations.

IKEDA • In a report on the relations between cancer deaths among Americans and various risk factors, the epidemiologist Dr. Richard Doll of Oxford University stated that diet is involved in 35% and smoking in 30% of cancer cases. The two together account for 65%—well over half—of all cases of cancer leading to death in the United States.

This prompted Takeshi Hirayama, director of the Japanese National Cancer Center Research Institute, to say that modification of life style and habits—eating and smoking—makes it possible to keep cancer in check. The most commonly consulted cancer prevention guide in Japan, issued by the Japanese National Cancer Center, is called "Twelve Measures for Cancer Prevention" (see Chart 1).

The American Association for Cancer Research published a similar guide entitled "Nutrition and Cancer." Explaining the importance of diet and eating habits in cancer prevention, the American report recommends controlling obesity, reducing overall fat intake, and eating large quantities of fibrous foods. Many of these recommendations are identical to the guidelines advocated in Japan as well.

Green and yellow vegetables, no tobacco, a balanced and regular life style

SIMARD • As I said earlier, certain organic substances are believed to be possible causes of cancer. Primary prevention consists in applying measures to counteract their action. The Japanese National Cancer Center's "Twelve Measures for Cancer Prevention" covers all the important steps to be taken within the framework of primary prevention. It correctly emphasizes the influence of diet and smoking—both the effects of smoking on smokers and second-hand smoke on others.

The first epidemiological studies showing that the dietary regimen can play a role in cancer began appearing in the sixties, and their numbers have grown rapidly ever since. There are now many well-documented studies dealing with the effects of diet on breast cancer; cancer of the digestive tract, the endometrium, and the prostate gland; and laryngeal, pharyngeal, and many other types of cancer. Nonetheless, even though some studies suggest that certain kinds of diet or certain consumer products either reduce or increase the risk of cancer, the evidence is still contradictory, and viewpoints continue to diverge sharply about conclusions that can be drawn.

Many of these studies deal with food additives. It is estimated that about 2,500 substances are added to foods, by chance or deliberately, to improve flavor, color, or appearance. This opens an enormous field for research since it takes years of study to prove that a substance is harmless.

CHART 1

Twelve Measures for Cancer Prevention

1. Eat a varied and balanced diet.
2. Do not eat the same foods too frequently.
3. Avoid overeating.
4. Avoid excessive consumption of alcohol.
5. Reduce tobacco consumption.
6. Eat a variety of foods containing sufficient amounts of vitamins A, C, and E and fiber.
7. Limit salty foods and avoid very hot foods.
8. Avoid charred or burnt food.
9. Never eat food that has been exposed to mold.
10. Avoid excessive exposure to direct sunlight.
11. Avoid overwork.
12. Maintain good personal cleanliness habits.

Powerful communications media like the press, radio, and television inform the public of the existence of these problems. Consumer associations popping up practically everywhere demand product quality guarantees. The public now knows that foods may contain toxic substances and that food additives may have carcinogenic properties. Still, little is known about these properties, because new substances are continually appearing on the market and because experimentation on each new product is time-consuming and expensive.

IKEDA • Yes, I can see how difficult that must be.

SIMARD • As well as leading to obesity, arteriosclerosis, and cardiac infarction, a high-fat diet is conducive to cancer of the digestive tract. People would be well-advised to follow the recommendations of nutritionists, who suggest that fats should constitute no more than 30% of the daily food ration. We must get used to eating much less fat. In Western countries, fats account for more than 40% of caloric intake.

Finally, Dr. Dennis P. Burkitt, a noted British physician, has recently drawn our attention to the importance of a greater dietary intake of cellulose as a good means of defense against colon and rectal cancer.

In spite of the absence of conclusive proof, increased intake of raw vegetables and raw fruit is generally recommended for the same reason.

Early detection and overcoming fear of death

IKEDA • In terms of early detection, the Japanese system of cancer examination is said to be the best in the world. In particular, examinations for early detection of stomach and uterine cancer produce reliable results. The Japanese Cancer Association's "Ten Warning Signs" are a good example of the kind of efforts being expended (see Chart 2).

CHART 2

Ten Warning Signs

1. Has the patient lost weight, become wan or pale in appearance, or developed anemia without apparent cause or specific particular discomfort?
   (ALL TYPES OF CANCER)

2. Are there persistent sores or ulcers in the mouth or on the skin that do not heal normally?
   (CANCER OF THE TONGUE, SKIN CANCER)

3. Is the voice hoarse for prolonged periods?
   (LARYNGEAL CANCER)

4. Does the patient have a persistent cough and bloody phlegm?
   (LUNG CANCER)

5. Does food seem to stay in the throat when it is swallowed?
   (CANCER OF THE ESOPHAGUS)

6. Does the patient suffer from persistent stomach pain or loss of appetite?
   (STOMACH CANCER)

7. Are bowel movements and stool normal? Is there blood in the stool?
   (CANCER OF THE LARGE INTESTINE)

8. Are there one or more persistent lumps in the breast?
   (BREAST CANCER)

9. Is there unusual or increased vaginal discharge, possibly containing blood? Is there unusual or bloody discharge upon physical contact?
   (UTERINE CANCER)

10. Is it difficult to urinate? Does the urine contain blood?
    (PROSTATE AND LIVER CANCER)

SIMARD · I agree that, as guidelines for early detection and diagnosis (secondary prevention) of cancer, the "Ten Warning Signs" cover the essentials. The Canadian Cancer Society makes similar recommendations. The fact that both organizations see things the same way reinforces the theory that early detection reduces the sickness and mortality rates of all kinds of cancer.

I personally think that programs aimed at cancer prevention should be more broadly applied. Primary prevention is far preferable to diagnosis—even early diagnosis. Still, early diagnosis makes it possible to avoid therapeutic methods that are costly and invasive, as well as physically debilitating.

IKEDA · The Japanese physician Hiro'omi Kono has published data on the main reasons that cancer often progresses to the point where it is difficult or impossible to treat before patients consult physicians. Some of the results of his work are included in Chart 3.

His survey of 50 patients with terminal gastric cancer showed that patients did not delay diagnosis because they were too busy at work, although I suspect that they may have waited until their jobs started to suffer, but because—and this is the crux of the matter—they were overconfident in their own good health. They chose to ignore the signals their own bodies were sending them. Furthermore, because of poor communication, family members paid little attention to each other's health and overlooked physical warning signs that seemed only minor.

CHART 3

Reasons for Delayed Cancer Diagnosis

- ☐ Though aware of cancer-like symptoms, the patient chooses to interpret them on his or her own and fails to seek medical examination. **(70%)**
- ☐ The members of the family communicate poorly, fail to suggest a medical examination and contribute to the patient's procrastination. **(50%)**
- ☐ The patient is too busy at work to take the time to see a doctor. **(30%)**

Psychologists describe a situation in which subconscious fear of death from cancer causes people to dull their sensibility to their own mental and physical abnormalities. Early and effective diagnosis and treatment depend on the way people perceive and react to cancer. Individuals must realize that cancer is not always fatal, and they must cultivate the life-force needed to overcome a groundless fear of dying. At the same time, people must learn about their bodies, observe them scrupulously and develop the determination to react quickly to problems. Another vital point, to my mind, is that family members sincerely care for each other and reinforce mutual bonds of affection and trust.

SIMARD • I must agree. Psychological factors play a terribly important role in cancer. This is true for healthy people as well as for cancer patients. The mere word *cancer* immediately evokes images of death, incurable disease, solitude, abandonment, and powerlessness.

Throughout the history of our species, all kinds of diseases thought to be incurable have threatened human life. Down the ages, leprosy (Hansen's disease), the plague, tuberculosis, and many other sicknesses have endangered populations large and small. Until very recently, no one—including scientists—understood their causes, much less their treatment. No one had the least idea of how to limit the ravages they caused.

Although AIDS currently rivals cancer as a medical scourge, combining the same connotation of incurability with that of a just chastisement for a reprehensible life style, cancer—with its adjective *malignant*—still has the monopoly on being associated with infernal images. As a metaphor of evil, *cancer* is now used in economic and political language: unemployment is described as a cancer of society, and terrorism as a cancer of democracy.

Chemotherapy, surgery, and radiation

IKEDA • Though once thought hopeless, today pulmonary tuberculosis is almost entirely curable. Do you believe that one day we will find a medicine that can completely cure cancer?

SIMARD • Cancer has long been regarded as incurable. As long as its cause is unknown, any disease remains sinister and mysterious and generates physical and psychological dread of contagion. I have heard of hospitals in some parts of the world that, blinded by such fears, refuse to admit cancer patients.

For viral infections, effective drugs can be developed by studying the virus itself. But we are still in the dark on cancer. We cannot develop drugs to counteract the disease at its source simply because we do not know what the source is. The unfortunate reality is that right now effective medicines and therapies to cure cancer are still a long way off.

As I said earlier, however, chemotherapy has proven very effective in treating juvenile cancer. Today, 90 to 95% of all childhood leukemia (blood cancer) can be cured.

IKEDA • That is certainly very encouraging.

SIMARD • Chemotherapy is still new. It was born of pharmacological research on poison gases produced during World War II. Another noteworthy advance, also dating from the early 1940s, was the discovery by a Canadian named Huggins (1901–97) that estrogen can be used to treat prostate cancer. Huggins received a Nobel Prize for this discovery.

IKEDA • What is your specialty, Dr. Simard? Could you describe your own research for us in concrete terms that we non-specialists can understand?

SIMARD • That is relatively easy. My research concentrates on how to use anticancer agents to fight cancer cells. I am also trying to discover how viruses create cancer in animals and humans.

IKEDA • The side effect of anticancer drugs is that they cause suffering by destroying not only cancerous cells, but normal cells as well. Your research, I believe, aims to overcome this drawback.

SIMARD • Yes. Certain antibodies, called monoclonal antibodies, recognize cancer cells exclusively. If these antibodies can be administered in association with an anticancer drug, the drug acts only on cancer cells, with no effect on normal cells.

There is still a lot of work remaining to make cancer drugs more effective, that is, to ensure that the vector—the monoclonal antibody, in this case—selects only cancer cells with consistency and precision. Advances in this area hold incalculable potential for cancer therapy.

IKEDA • I gather that radiation therapy, too, is making rapid strides. How effective are such treatments as cobalt 60?

SIMARD • Radiation therapies have proven effective against some types of cancer, but they can only reduce the volume of cancerous cells; they are still unable to eliminate them entirely.

To treat some kinds of cancer, it is necessary to prescribe radiotherapy and medicinal therapy in addition to surgery. This method of associative therapy translates into a constant increase in survival rates. Cases of permanent remission, too, occur, especially in patients 30 and over.

Using two or three therapies together makes great progress possible in the battle against this illness. But because of the high level of technology, skill, and expertise such treatment requires and the inevitable recourse to expensive drugs not always readily available, it is hard to determine whether the new therapeutic methods can be used successfully on a worldwide scale.

Effects of the emotional state on immunity

IKEDA • I understand that immunotherapy is being studied as a way of inhibiting cancer. Naturally, this would involve the body's natural defenses against illness, of which the immune system is the most important. What exactly is the role of white blood cells and lymphocytes within the immune system?

SIMARD • All vertebrates are equipped with defensive capacities— immune response—to protect them from micro-organisms and other pathogenic agents that cause diseases of various kinds. Because of these defenses, we are able to withstand and recover from a vast assortment of infectious diseases. The body's natural defense capability is an important topic in medical science. Physicians and scientists in cancer research believe it offers a valid defense against the disease. According to their line of reasoning, if the human body cannot avoid cancer, perhaps there is a way to limit its consequences by taking advantage of natural immunity.

Essentially, the immune system is based on two types of cells found in lymphoid tissue and disseminated throughout the human body.

B cells, the first type, manufacture antibodies. Antibodies are clusters of proteins in the blood. There are several thousand different kinds, each one programmed to attach to an antigen. Antigens, for their part, stimulate the formation of antibodies.

The T cell, or T lymphocyte, is the second type. These white blood cells, formed in lymphoid tissue, make certain that the immune defense system functions as planned. They circulate through the bloodstream on constant patrol for antigens.

Whenever antigens are spotted, the immune system stores the information in its data bank. As soon as the same antigens reappear, the immune system identifies them and launches a counterattack. Once they have detected antigens, sensitized lymphocytes can transmit that information to other cells. Thus, when the right conditions conjoin, lymphocytes can mobilize a massive immune response.

IKEDA • Would you say, then, that by energizing the action of lymphocytes, we could control the proliferation of cancerous cells?

SIMARD • If, indeed, the immune system can eliminate cancerous cells, then the key to preventing the development of cancerous tumors would be to stimulate an immune-system reaction. Inversely, it could be that cancerous cells develop and cancer progresses precisely when the immune system is not working correctly.

IKEDA • How far has research advanced in this area?

SIMARD • So far, progress has been a bit slow, and we are not certain precisely which directions will be most productive and beneficial. But there can be no doubt that stimulating the immune response is a valid therapeutic avenue. In cases of AIDS, the immune system has broken down. AIDS patients are very vulnerable to infectious diseases and often develop cancer. It may be concluded, therefore, that strengthening immunity prevents the emergence of cancer.

IKEDA • Where is the most advanced research in immunology going on now?

SIMARD • In the United States probably, but nobody can predict where a major breakthrough will occur.

IKEDA • Reports in the field of psychosomatic medicine about strengthening immunity claim that emotions like happiness, gratitude, hope, and satisfaction enliven lymphocytic action, whereas suffering, anger, resentment, sadness, and so on dampen it.

A very interesting article called "Does Spiritual Healing in Cancer Prolong Life?" by Dr. David Spiegel[1] describes an investigation conducted on 109 breast cancer patients. The subjects were divided into two groups, only one of which received spiritual therapy. Results showed that patients who received spiritual therapy regained emotional and psychological stability. The length of time before death and the survival rates were twice as great in the spiritual-therapy group. In other words, the report acknowledged the effect of spiritual healing on longevity. Although its mechanism is a topic for future research, surely this indicates that spiritual condition affects the immune system.

According to the Buddhist principle of "oneness of body and mind (*shikishin-funi*)," the physical aspect and the mental or spiritual aspect are two facets of a single entity—literally "two but not two." At the same time, although these two aspects are united and inseparable on the most basic level, they fall into two different spheres of phenomena.

So if, as I believe, the body and the spirit influence each other so extensively, it follows that joy, hope and other positive sentiments activate physiological mechanisms and reinforce the body's immune powers, whereas despair and other negative sentiments weaken them.

SIMARD • From a strictly scientific point of view, I must say that it is exceedingly difficult to design and carry out psychosomatic laboratory tests to establish a clear correlation between human psychology and disease. I would hasten to add, however, that in the case of cardiovascular diseases, evidence shows that emotions like joy and anguish are definitely related to health and sickness.

Cancer, too, can be brought on by stress, as the term "stress cancer" indicates. Specialists in cancer research should remain broad-minded enough to entertain all these theories and possibilities.

1. *The Lancet*. New York. October 1989.

Signs of correlation between cancer and emotions

IKEDA • Josei Toda, my mentor, used to tell us that the human body is like a compact but highly diversified pharmaceutical plant. The endocrine glands secrete all kinds of hormones, while endorphins in the brain act as natural painkillers. The body produces white blood cells that combat disease-causing bacteria and enzymes that affect chemical reactions. If we look at the body in this light, there is a lot of truth in Toda's metaphor.

SIMARD • The idea of the body as a pharmaceutical plant is very unusual. The brain is known to secrete endorphins, sometimes called internal morphine. Acupuncture, the fulcrum of oriental medicine, is presumed to accelerate endorphin secretion.

Joggers, for instance, sometimes feel buoyantly invigorated and fatigue-free. Very probably this sensation can be attributed to endorphins. Anger, on the other hand, has the effect of increasing adrenaline secretion, with a corresponding rise in blood-pressure and bronchial dilation.

IKEDA • According to the ideas of psychosomatic medicine, people without hope or a reason to live and people who torment themselves with insecurity and repressed anger are susceptible to cancer. In contrast, people who can discover fresh reasons for living and people who are strong-willed and goal-oriented have the strength to resist cancer. What do you think of such opinions?

SIMARD • It is very interesting to consider the genesis of cancer from a psychological standpoint. Patients are always concerned by the diagnosis, and they may be anxious about the gravity of their condition, but reactions vary widely from person to person. The possibility of an amputation—of a leg or a breast for instance—causes much anxiety about the perceived "maiming" of the body. People also worry about being saddled with a permanent surgical orifice. Many fear that their lives will change radically after treatment. When no therapy succeeds, they imagine an endless struggle made still more unbearable by the emotional burden which inevitably grows heavier with time.

Depending on the gravity of the illness, the patient may be forced to give up work for a long time or, in certain cases, never really return to normal life, even after rehabilitation. Some people end up withdrawing from active social involvement and live out their lives in profound depression.

IKEDA • In connection with this topic, too, Dr. Hiro'omi Kono's data are relevant (see Chart 4).

According to his report, drawn-out depression or the loss of a purpose in living causes cancer cells to increase and spread faster, retarding convalescence. But a strong will that discovers new reasons to live and moves forward optimistically causes cancer cells to degenerate. All over the world, the relationship between cancer and the mental state is being pathologically and statistically researched.

CHART 4

Psychological/Emotional Factors and Cancer Patients

1. People who have a very unhappy childhood may be more susceptible to cancer.

2. People who experience serious stress before the onset of illness, such as personal bereavement (death of a spouse or a child), experience shock and grief followed by despair and loss of the will to live.

3. Cancer patients generally appear to be well adapted socially, but in fact they are inwardly maladjusted and tend to be self-repressive.

4. Cancer patients have a strong tendency to inflict on themselves the tensions, anxiety, anger and other emotions they have trouble expressing.

SIMARD • Suggestions that some people are at higher risk for cancer or that mental stress and overwork encourage cancer could be important clues for future research to follow. The possibility was entertained in the distant past. Almost two millennia ago, the second-century Greek physician Galen (ca. 129–ca. 200 BCE) observed that melancholy or depressed women were more prone to breast cancer. But to tell the truth, research in this area has made little progress over the centuries. It is very difficult to produce hard evidence of a clear relationship between psychological states and cancer.

Still, although there is no irrefutable proof of the psychological effect, it is useful to include a psychiatrist or a psychologist in the therapeutic group to prevent certain psychological drifts that cancer can cause. Doctors and nurses try hard to pay special attention to the psychological difficulties associated with cancer, but they are still unable to handle these problems completely. Eager for training in this area, they are doing their best to learn about the psychological aspects of cancer therapy.

The body's constant countermeasures

IKEDA • Dr. Kono's data make it clear that a large number of cancer patients (about one-third) have experienced the loneliness and unhappiness of losing one or both parents or some other loved one during childhood, suggesting that this experience becomes a psychological stressor that later triggers the onset of cancer. This makes me think that of all kinds of stress, the loss of a loved one has the greatest impact.

It seems to me, however, that a child orphaned at an early age but surrounded by people embodying unshakeable motherly and fatherly support and care could be free of psychological stress and able to rally the internal powers needed to combat cancer cells.

The idea of such an "unshakeable" presence, with its inherent fatherly and motherly overtones, is reminiscent of the role of philosophy or, even more so, religion. Is it possible that, through religion, an individual could undergo an existential conversion and draw from this experience the vibrant life force needed to successfully combat cancer? It seems perfectly fitting to me that philosophy and religion should play a vital role in fighting cancer.

SIMARD • If we study a group of cancer patients and observe that they have personality problems, it becomes impossible to overlook the influence somatic sickness—cancer in this case—has exerted on their mental behavior. Furthermore, because no personality analysis was performed before the onset of sickness, it is impossible to eliminate the inverse proposition.

It is often possible to identify in a patient's personal history a stressful event shortly before the first symptoms of illness. But can we attribute a triggering nature to such stress? Personally, I am not ready to take that step. Many stresses do not translate into serious illness—cancer. Moreover, the evaluation of stress is highly subjective.

IKEDA • I see what you mean. People may experience the same kind of stress, but their organism's response will differ according to how that stress is overcome.

A person may be defeated by stress or use it as a life-reinforcing power. In the latter case, I think an existential conversion occurs.

SIMARD • Of course, this is one track to explore. Owing to the difficulties of differing interpretations and the absence of evidence and experimental models, however, we are still a long way from any kind of certitude.

IKEDA • In a dialogue I conducted some years ago with Norman Cousins (1915–90),[2] who was called the "conscience of America" for his compassion in advocating treatment for Japanese victims of American A-bomb radiation, he expressed the view that the human being is endowed with a healing system and a system of convictions. Mr. Cousins believed that the two work together to cure illness. I, too, believe that human life has an innate capacity to overcome disease.

SIMARD • Frankly, I also think that the body is constantly manufacturing something new to fight against malignant growths that affect it internally.

IKEDA • Coming from someone with many years' experience in cancer research, your words carry a great weight of hope and courage for many people.

3. Cancer and Disclosure: The Doctor-Patient Bond

Human dignity and disclosure

IKEDA • Let's turn now to informing the patient of the diagnosis. Should doctors inform patients of cancer diagnoses? Since the kind of treatment depends in part on whether the doctor chooses to tell the patient, this is an extremely important decision. Specialist groups

---

2. *Sekai Shimin no Taiwa – A Dialogue Toward Global Harmonization*. Tokyo: The Mainichi Newspapers. 1991.

in Japan have been adopting an increasingly positive attitude toward disclosure, which seems to be becoming the prevailing trend.

The sufferings caused by cancer fall into three main categories. First is physical pain. Particularly in advanced and terminal cases, severe, continuous pain can result in the loss of human dignity. Second is the anxiety and fear associated with the disruption or breakdown of social and personal life related to family, work, position, and property. Third is anxiety about and fear of death itself.

In the Buddhist view, there are three dimensions of human suffering: physical pain (*ku-ku*), spiritual, mental and social anguish related to family and society (*e-ku*), and existential agony or fear of death (*gyo-ku*). Overcoming these sufferings is the focus of debate on whether and how to inform cancer patients of their condition.

In many instances in Japan, cancer patients are still not informed. In Europe and the United States, on the other hand, disclosure is made in almost all instances. A survey conducted in 1973 by the *Journal of the American Medical Association* reported that 98% of physicians in the United States inform patients when they have cancer. Conceivably these divergent approaches reflect differences between Japanese and Western views of life and death.

Protection of patients' rights accounts for the prevalence of disclosure in the West. The principle of informed consent means that patients have the right to know and select their own therapy.

Quality of life is another consideration. It is believed that merely extending life is insufficient. To enable patients to live their remaining lives in as fulfilled a way as possible by giving them care that respects their humanity, disclosure of the nature of their condition is essential. In addition, in places like the United States, where medical malpractice suits are frequent, disclosure may help provide verifying evidence in the event of court battles.

Japanese doctors, however, are concerned that the shock of disclosure could plunge their patient into a profound depression and accelerate death. They believe that they can help patients die in peace by leaving them uninformed. More recently, however, attitudes have been changing, and apparently more and more doctors are opting for disclosure.

SIMARD · You have brought up some crucial points about disclosure in the case of cancer patients. And clearly Buddhism makes a valuable contribution to the debate. In my opinion, patients have the right to know everything about the state of their health. Besides, when they are well informed, they are generally more cooperative and amenable to the treatments judged most advisable. My own experience and that of my colleagues confirm this.

For personal reasons, some patients do not wish to know the truth about the state of their health. They are ill-inclined to ask questions about the diagnosis, and doctors should respect their feelings. Often their initial resistance weakens, though, and they come to want to know about their condition. Personally, if I had cancer, I would want to know.

IKEDA · As a scientist, you are prepared to observe your own condition coolly and objectively. Actually, with the side effects of modern radiation treatment and anticancer drugs, the truth would be hard to conceal.

SIMARD · Patients know more about their own physical condition than others think.

IKEDA · As you say, knowing the truth about their illness may make patients more receptive to treatment and it probably deepens the patient-doctor bond. Another advantage is that knowing that their days are numbered may stimulate people to complete unfinished tasks and life-long undertakings. It may give them the impetus to spend time with their family and friends. Most of all, confrontation with one's own death can inspire awareness of the limits of life and turn the mind toward eternal things.

When it comes to disclosure of cancer diagnoses, I think the following things should be carefully considered. First, the need for mutual trust between the doctors and medical-care staff, and between the doctor and the patient. Second, the need to establish a highly qualified medical team. Third, the importance of encouraging the patient to combat the disease. Fourth, the importance of support from family and friends. Fifth, the importance, for the patient, of adopting a vision of mortal life and a philosophy of life and death.

Carelessly performed, disclosure can generate severe anxiety and depression, even leading to suicide. It can deprive the patient of the will to continue treatment, thus causing further physical weakening. In some cases, it may bring a halt to all the patient's social activities.

Hope and the innate capacity to defeat illness

SIMARD • Once we recognize the patient's right to be informed and the doctor's duty to transmit this information, the thorny question of how to communicate the nature and severity of the sickness remains. It is important not only to reveal the diagnosis to the patient, but also to explain it to family and friends. This assumes the doctor knows the family, who will provide indispensable psychological support to the patient and help him or her cope with the sickness. The number of meetings needed and the suitability of allowing others to be present at the disclosure must be determined on the basis of the patient's age and personality, and the availability of family members.

IKEDA • That is extremely valuable and practical advice. The final chapter of life is subject to various kinds of suffering—called the sufferings of death or *shiku* in Buddhist terms. The heart of the disclosure problem is whether people can overcome these sufferings and attain tranquility. Positive aspects must be sought, and seen to outweigh negative aspects. Suffering—physical or other—must be eliminated. They must be transformed from pain to comfort. Because illness and condition vary from patient to patient, decisions must be made on a case-by-case basis.

SIMARD • No matter what doctors say to their patients, they must always take the patients' age and intellectual and cultural background into consideration when deciding the best way to communicate the information. They must use simple language without the gobbledygook of medical jargon. They would be well advised to ask the patients and their families to repeat back to them what they have just explained, to prevent unjustified fears and misinterpretations.

IKEDA • Yes. Explaining the disease in a way the patient can fully understand is essential. One Buddhist sutra uses an expression that means "pleasing words" or "love words," where the word *love* means altruistic, philanthropic compassion. The passage in the *Epidamo jiyimenzu lun* (The Abhidharma Verse Commentary on the Recitation

Teaching) reads, "What are these love words like? They give pleasure, they are pleasant and moving. They are pronounced with tenderness and soft glances." The same passage exhorts people not to use "words that make people frown." I think that patients find what they are told easier to accept when the message is couched in such "love words."

SIMARD • I can only agree with you. As you said earlier, Mr. Ikeda, in communicating with people committed to their care, doctors must seize every occasion to encourage them and reinforce their hope of survival. Trust in the doctor and faith in the treatment greatly enhance chances of triumphing over the suffering caused by the sickness. The patient who entertains firm hope bears up better under anxiety and pain.

IKEDA • Very aptly put. Hope provides the driving force to challenge the diverse hardships of life, including the suffering of disease.

During our discussions together, Dr. Martin Seligman (1942–), president of the American Psychological Association, called hope the key to overcoming suffering and living optimistically.

In *Man's Search for Meaning: Experiences in the Concentration Camp* (1947), the Austrian psychoanalyst Dr. Viktor E. Frankl (1905–97) wrote that he survived a Nazi concentration camp not because he was in good health, but because he consistently believed in the future and went on hoping. He said that those who abandoned hope soon collapsed inwardly and died. He attributed to hope the power to strengthen the body and prolong life. In a similar vein, the Buddhist scripture known as *Abhidharma Kosha Shastra* (A Treasury of Analyses of the Law) says "Hope nurtures the body and prolongs life."

SIMARD • That is absolutely true.

IKEDA • To achieve good results in cancer disclosure, tests and examinations or treatment, strong bonds of trust between physicians and medical staff and patients and families are essential.

The urgency of restoring human bonds

SIMARD • The intrusion of anonymous "invaders" between doctor and patient constitutes a relatively new medical problem. By invaders I mean devices, instruments, and an ever-increasing battery of tests and equipment. Nowadays, before they ever see the face of a doctor, outpatients see a multitude of machines.

IKEDA • How right you are!

SIMARD • You are ushered into an examination room where blood samples are taken and x-ray, chemical, and other tests performed. Of course all these tests are valuable—they provide the doctor with the data needed to make the diagnosis. But being satisfied with tests hinders the formation of necessary bonds between doctor and patient.

IKEDA • The very thought of medical examinations is enough to keep many people away from hospitals.

SIMARD • Yet these invaders are the fruit of the very technological breakthroughs that now make it possible to cure patients who, only yesterday, were considered hopeless. Nonetheless, they threaten the close, privileged bond that is so vital between physician and patient. Precisely because this bond has become so fragile, we must work all the harder to avoid neglecting the human factor in the healing process.

IKEDA • That is a very important point. As medicine advances, we must strive to ensure that it becomes, not more mechanical, but more humane. After all, medicine exists for the sake of humanity.

SIMARD • True. And doctors themselves certainly have no easy role. They must earn a living, and at the same time enormous social pressure compels them to call upon the newest medical technology. Still, this cannot justify neglecting to build a sound rapport with their patients.

No device—no machine, no high-tech tools—should intervene in a way that excludes the human factor. I firmly believe that medical-school curricula must be revised to provide theoretical and practical training in doctor-patient relations.

IKEDA • Hippocrates envisioned the physician as a treasury of useful suggestions. He said that physicians should learn to generate a lively and comforting atmosphere, because solemnity and severity distance the healthy and the ill alike. There is no question that meeting with an aloof, self-important, punctilious doctor can be upsetting. Hippocrates advised making the doctor's and the patient's chairs the same height. Don't look down on people in distress, he warned. Regard them as your equals, and regard them with compassion.

SIMARD • The doctor-patient relationship must be thoroughly reviewed and restructured. This is an issue that concerns all members of the medical profession.

IKEDA • Yes, I can understand why. We must restore the human bond. Like Hippocrates, Shakyamuni described the ideal physician as brimming with true humanity. For instance, a passage in the *Sovereign Kings of the Golden Light Sutra* instructs physicians to approach ill people with compassion and without greedy thoughts of personal profit.

One especially interesting aspect of Buddhist ideas on medicine is the emphasis laid on the patient's wisdom. *The Great Canon of Monastic Rules* urges people to learn and to expand their knowledge, to think independently and to use their wisdom and their knowledge for the sake of their own health.

SIMARD • All of us must think seriously about ways of informing and educating the public. In all countries, a gap separates the informed from the uninformed—those who can read and judge with a critical eye news of scientific discoveries and those who lack the basic knowledge to understand and assess what is happening in science and technology. As a result of this ignorance, many are led to blindly accept the effectiveness of any old treatment or find themselves refusing chances to receive a treatment that might help them. The outcome is too many unfortunate victims of unscrupulous charlatans.

IKEDA • No one should be victimized by greedy frauds. People need wisdom and common sense to avoid being taken advantage of.

SIMARD • In this day and age, if we want to preserve the human element in life, we must make certain that more people can analyze and discuss scientific and social problems.

IKEDA • It certainly appears that the best elements of human nature are being lost. Success is measured in other terms. Listen to this Quebecois poet, Felix Leclerc (1914–88), "Among so many hands / Trying to deprive you of everything / How beautiful is the single hand / Reaching out to give you something." In this highly materialist era, most people seem almost wholly bent on profiting from others. In the midst of so many grabbing hands, the single, giving hand is all the more radiant. I hope this dialogue—by raising awareness— will be seen as a "giving hand."

4. AIDS—Menace and Countermeasures

The origins of AIDS

IKEDA • Following your suggestion, Dr. Simard, we will now take up the vital issue of acquired immune deficiency syndrome, or AIDS. During the late twentieth century, AIDS became an inimical enemy to humanity and in all likelihood it will continue to threaten lives well into the twenty-first century.

SIMARD • Yes, you are right. AIDS may prove to be the greatest calamity of the new century.

IKEDA • When were the first occurrences of AIDS reported?

SIMARD • In the early 1980s, AIDS first appeared as an infectious disease previously unknown in the United States.

In the winter of 1981, doctors in California and New York were surprised to observe occurrences of such relatively uncommon ailments as pneumonia caused by a protozoan organism (*pneumocystis carinii*) and Kaposi's sarcoma, an infrequently occurring skin cancer. Strangely enough, in all cases, the patients were men in their thirties, formerly in excellent health, with only one thing in common: homosexuality. From that time on, however, they shared another characteristic: the collapse of their immune system. Incidentally, these rare ailments can also be associated with an immune-system deficiency imputable to, for instance, certain genetic diseases or the immuno-suppressive treatments that inevitably accompany organ transplants or chemotherapy.

Upon learning of these findings in 1981, the Center for Disease Control in Atlanta, Georgia, published a report constituting the first alarm signal. Within three months, some hundred analogous cases had been reported, mostly in New York and San Francisco. When their immune systems collapsed, the relatively young patients, almost all homosexuals, were stricken with such so-called opportunistic infections as mycoses of the oral cavity or esophagus, or even aggressive, ulcerous forms of herpes. The conclusion was self-evident: we were dealing with an epidemic of a type totally unknown till then. It was dubbed acquired immune deficiency syndrome or AIDS.

IKEDA • At first, because homosexuals were the only people infected, the sickness was thought to be a rare disease limited to them. We shall deal with prejudice and discrimination against AIDS patients later, but the appearance of any disease of unknown origin can trigger extreme reactions of social panic.

Was it in 1983 that the AIDS virus was first identified?

SIMARD • That year, the laboratories of Professors Luc Montagnier (1932–) and Robert Gallo (1937–) identified a retrovirus as the cause of AIDS. This virus is now known as the human immunodeficiency virus (HIV). Two years later, a test was developed to detect the presence of the virus in blood.

I should add that one of the characteristics of the AIDS epidemic is our current knowledge of two types or strains of HIV with different epidemiological profiles. Whereas HIV–1 is the principal cause of the epidemic in America and the Caribbean, two strains—HIV–1 and HIV–2—are prevalent in different parts of Africa.

IKEDA • What about the origin of the AIDS virus? Did it exist before it manifested itself in humans? What do you think of the theory that AIDS is indigenous to Africa?

SIMARD • As for the origin of the disease, we believe that it appeared at about the same time in Africa and the United States. The precise origin of HIV is unknown. Rumors claimed that it was the product of a laboratory experiment as part of the development of some sort of genetic therapy, but that hypothesis has been abandoned. It now seems most probable that HIV emerged during the last few decades somewhere in Central Africa. Actually, HIV contamination has been traced back to serum collected from Ugandan children in 1972 and 1973. This indicates that the virus existed in an endemic state in a rural population in Central Africa at that time.

Retroviruses very similar to HIV have also been isolated in African green monkeys. This is why the virus is thought to have mutated suddenly to become pathogenic in human beings. It could therefore have been present in humans for years without causing AIDS. Or it could have caused many cases of AIDS that went unrecognized because the syndrome was still undefined.

Opportunistic infection and modes of transmission

IKEDA • How exactly is the disease transmitted?

SIMARD • The currently proven ways AIDS is transmitted are sexual transmission (homosexual or heterosexual), which is the most common; transmission through HIV-contaminated syringes; transmission from an infected mother to her infant during pregnancy, delivery, or breastfeeding; and transmission through blood transfusions of HIV-contaminated blood or blood products.

IKEDA • In Japan, a few years ago, infection of hemophiliacs through HIV-contaminated blood products caused a great uproar.

SIMARD • Of the four major ways the disease can be transmitted, the most common, worldwide, is sexual intercourse. Research to date indicates that contagion through air, water, or food is virtually nil. The disease is transmitted only when the virus enters the body through a contaminated needle or blood product or through direct exchange of bodily fluids with an HIV carrier.

IKEDA • In other words, ordinary contact with HIV carriers or AIDS patients in daily life entails absolutely no risk of infection?

SIMARD • None at all. It is eminently important to understand this.

IKEDA • Accurate information generates responses that can prevent the spread of contamination and eliminate groundless fears, enabling people to live confidently with HIV carriers and AIDS patients.

SIMARD • Without a doubt. Public ignorance about AIDS is a more serious menace than the disease itself.

IKEDA • What kinds of symptoms develop from HIV infection? Are there symptoms peculiar to AIDS?

SIMARD • HIV almost exclusively attacks the T4 lymphocytes, which play an essential role in the immune system specific to the organism. These lymphocytes carry on their surfaces a protein called CD4, a kind of cell keyhole to which HIV has the key. Once inside the cell, the virus can remain quiet for several months, during which seroconversion takes place. This process generally takes from six to eight weeks after introduction of HIV into the organism. Most of the time, this initial phase of infection is free of symptoms, but routine blood tests can detect it. In some cases, however, infected persons demonstrate flu-like symptoms, including fever, headaches, muscular pain, and glandular disorders.

IKEDA • How long does it take for the HIV-infected patient to develop AIDS symptoms?

SIMARD • There is a second phase which may last up to five years and during which a variety of things may occur. Sometimes we observe asymptomatic forms that evolve over a long period. With more than ten years of hindsight, we now know that all infected individuals eventually contract AIDS and that, even though they may remain free of symptoms themselves for years, they are nonetheless capable of transmitting the virus.

We may also see minor forms of infection, depending on the extent of multiplication and dissemination of the virus, that manifest themselves by general signs: high fever, weight loss, gastrointestinal troubles, and skin conditions. Strictly speaking, however, none of these signs is specific to AIDS.

IKEDA • What symptoms occur when AIDS has fully developed?

SIMARD • From the moment the infection leads to a serious immune deficiency, we witness a group of grave symptoms associated with either very particular infections or the development of cancerous tumors, of which Kaposi's sarcoma is the most widely known. The infections and tumors are not directly related to HIV—HIV is simply responsible for creating a favorable terrain for their development.

IKEDA • And this is why they are called opportunistic infections?

SIMARD • Yes. Normally many microbes—viruses, bacteria, fungi, and protozoa—inhabit our organism without creating problems, since our immune defense limits their numbers and prevents the full-scale invasions that are the source of illness.

As soon as our immune defenses weaken, these micro-organisms seize the opportunity to multiply actively. The numerous opportunistic infections associated with AIDS affect, above all, the lungs, the digestive tract, the nervous system and, less frequently, the skin. Often, these infections constitute the first pathological and revelatory expression of HIV infection. Among the most frequent and indicative infections brought on by AIDS are a form of pneumonia caused by a protozoan organism, *pneumocystis carinii*; a cytomegalovirus poly-visceral infection that can manifest itself as pneumonia, hepatitis, or encephalitis; and a herpes-simplex infection that provokes lesions of the skin or the mucous membranes.

These few examples of opportunistic infection illustrate the great complexity of symptoms that confront the doctor in the second phase of HIV infection. Still other equally serious symptoms that develop in the wake of HIV infection are called opportunistic cancers.

IKEDA • What are some of the main opportunistic cancers?

SIMARD • The most frequent is Kaposi's sarcoma, caused by the development of endothelial cells in the blood vessels of the skin, muscles, viscera, or ganglions. Other tumors composed of lymphoid tissue can develop after a serious breakdown of the immune system. These are malignant lymphomas originating in the lymphatic nodes. HIV does not cause these malignant tumors directly. By causing an immune deficiency, it simply opens the door for them.

Estimated HIV carriers and AIDS patients in 2000

IKEDA • In 1995, the number of HIV-infected people in the United States was reported to have reached one million. Today numbers of carriers in Africa and Southeast Asia are growing at an explosive rate. By some predictions, the number will reach forty million worldwide in the twenty-first century. What do you think, Dr. Simard?

SIMARD • When people talk of the galloping spread of HIV infection, they mean the exponential growth in the number of reported cases. The nature of AIDS and HIV infection makes statistics outmoded the moment they are published. From current observations, we estimate that, at the turn of the century, about 38 million people had been infected with HIV. Others think that a figure of 110 million constitutes a more realistic evaluation of the situation as it was in the year 2000.

IKEDA • Those are frightening figures. Do you think AIDS will continue to spread at this rate?

SIMARD • Clearly HIV-infection and the AIDS syndrome have reached pandemic proportions over the past decade. It is uncertain whether we can rapidly control or neutralize the pandemic because HIV is now endemic in the human population.

IKEDA • What can we do to check the spread of AIDS?

SIMARD • HIV is not highly contagious. Adequate preventive measures minimize its spread.

IKEDA • So prevention is the key to controlling this disease?

SIMARD • Exactly. Epidemiological data show that some people demonstrate a higher risk of HIV infection than the general population. For the moment, these people are essentially homosexuals and bisexuals; drug addicts using injectable substances; people with numerous sexual partners; people born or living in countries where infection is common and frequent; sexual partners of all these groups; and, of course, children born to infected mothers.

IKEDA • I know that drug addicts are a high-risk group. Their extreme poverty obliges them to share needles.

SIMARD • True. It is critically important to introduce preventive measures that, among other things, address problems of poverty and drug addiction. Educating high-risk groups is vital to checking the future spread of AIDS.

Variable virus: An obstacle to vaccine development

IKEDA • I understand just how crucial education can be when it comes to AIDS. Now I should like to discuss the different types of therapy currently being used to treat AIDS patients.

SIMARD • Treatment for AIDS is based on two totally different therapeutic methods, according to how far the syndrome has advanced. The first approach fights the virus and the infected cells to impede viral reproduction and eventually re-establish immunity. The second treats ailments promoted by immune deficiency—primarily opportunistic infections and cancers.

IKEDA • Can we look forward to the development of effective anti-AIDS medication?

SIMARD • One constraint is the scarcity of products that check the multiplication of viruses in general. We have at our disposal an arsenal of antibiotics and other drugs capable of dealing with bacterial infection, but viruses act differently. Viruses are, in effect, parasites that use cell metabolism to multiply. We can fight them only by considerably disturbing cellular metabolism, with the death of the host cell as a consequence. Clearly, that is not the desired goal. Antiviral treatment itself targets different phases of virus replication. The substances that have produced the best results to date call upon chemical structures that inhibit an enzyme (reverse transcriptase) responsible for viral reproduction.

IKEDA • Recently in Japan much attention has been devoted to Azidothymidine (AZT).

SIMARD • AZT treatment has demonstrated the ability to retard the reproduction of the virus considerably and, consequently, the manifestation of the sickness. Unfortunately, AZT becomes less effective after about one year of treatment. Its fairly serious side effects—nausea, headache, dizziness, and leucopoenia—require repeated control measures. This means frequent visits to enable the doctor in charge of treatment to closely observe the effects of the drug on the patient. Promising clinical trials are now being conducted to develop other drugs that inhibit the proteins the virus needs to multiply.

IKEDA • I understand that attempts are being made to develop a preventative vaccine.

SIMARD • In trying to develop a vaccine, we run up against numerous problems connected with the very nature and habits of this virus.

IKEDA • I know it is difficult, but could you explain simply what makes the AIDS virus so peculiar?

SIMARD • For one thing, the efficacy of a vaccine is directly proportional to the constancy of the virus. The AIDS virus varies greatly in terms of protein content and genome from patient to patient. The development of a vaccine to deal with one given viral structure runs the risk of failing to protect against other, slightly different structures.

IKEDA • I see. That must be a major obstacle to AIDS-vaccine development.

SIMARD • It is. For another thing, the virus can remain silent in the form of a provirus or can literally hide inside the central nervous system or in macrophages. Until now, this capability has prevented our finding a way to parry the viral strategy. Still, research in this area is very active and is oriented particularly toward using genetic engineering to manufacture a vaccine.

In any case, the development of an AIDS vaccine will undoubtedly be long and arduous. In the meantime, efforts are being made to find new methods of treatment like the so-called cocktail therapy, which uses a number of therapies simultaneously. I think we can expect progress in therapeutic techniques, even though we may have to wait.

5. AIDS and Human Rights

Prejudice based on misconceptions

IKEDA • Up to now we've been talking about the pathological nature of the threat AIDS poses to human life, but AIDS has other effects that are intimately involved with ethics and human rights. I should now like to call on Dr. Bourgeault to join us in broaching the topic of AIDS and human rights.

BOURGEAULT • As you say, AIDS raises questions of ethics and human rights that are today universal topics of debate.

IKEDA • AIDS highlights the need to build a society dedicated to human rights, and supporting human rights entails support for HIV-infected people. The dissemination of accurate information about the disease, research, the development of effective therapies and medicines, and respect for patients' rights are all very important.

To guard the rights of all human beings—including those affected by AIDS—first of all, we must break down barriers of prejudice and discrimination against HIV carriers.

BOURGEAULT • The stigmatization and discrimination of AIDS patients arise partly from the nature of the sickness, but even more from people's perceptions of it. When I think about the nature of the disease, I think of the apparently irreversible dynamic of its development, leading inescapably to death. We try all ways to avoid or at least retard the illness and death and, when that proves impossible, we gloss over the reality. AIDS patients—less so HIV-carriers than the physically afflicted—display the signs of sickness and of what I would call the universal human condemnation to death. I think that the mechanisms of AIDS transmission and latency make us fear—often mistakenly— being accidentally infected, perhaps without even knowing it.

Fortunately, as the apt title of the recent book *Maintenant que je ne vais plus mourir* (Now that I'm no longer going to die)[3] gives us to understand, new treatments are providing hope to the men and women who do daily battle against HIV within their own bodies.

IKEDA • Despite therapeutic advances being made, AIDS still entails the sufferings of illness and death. I admire all the noble efforts made to afford hope in the face of these primary sufferings.

BOURGEAULT • The prejudice against AIDS patients is nourished by erroneous perceptions and ideas about the sickness. People afflicted with AIDS and HIV carriers are victims twice over: they suffer physically from the disease and psychologically from social discrimination.

IKEDA • This makes it all the more urgent that accurate information about AIDS be disseminated. This is true in cases not only of sickness, but also of prejudices involving religion, philosophy, human rights, and many other issues. In this sense, dialogues such as the one we are conducting now are especially precious as a means of educating the public.

BOURGEAULT • In a sense, bias against AIDS patients is the product of prejudices and discriminatory attitudes. Even though the transmission mechanisms are well known—as Dr. Simard just explained—irrational fears persist. As if touching an infected person or even breathing the same air could cause contamination!

---

3. Manon Jourdenais, in collaboration with Jean-Guy Nadeau. *Maintenant que je ne vais plus mourir: L'expérience spirituelle d'homosexuels vivant avec le HIV/SIDA* (Now that I'm no longer going to die: The spiritual experience of homosexuals living with HIV/AIDS). Montreal: Fides. 1998.

It is not entirely coincidental that people have called AIDS a modern plague. The irrational fear, which leads to stigmatization and sometimes discrimination, arises because of the way the disease has been presented to the public. In Canada, associating the spread of the sickness with the arrival of immigrants, more specifically of Blacks, has awakened the old demons of racism. The sickness is also associated with sexual behavior that some consider reprehensible, even unnatural. These things partly explain why people do not always feel the kind of compassion toward AIDS patients that they otherwise spontaneously entertain for the sick. They also explain—once again in part—the stigmatization of AIDS patients.

IKEDA • Reports claim that in Japan some medical personnel often or even systematically refuse to treat people infected with HIV.

SIMARD • Attitudes toward people infected with HIV and AIDS vary considerably, ranging from disgust and fear to compassion and solidarity. This includes health professionals like doctors, dentists, and surgeons, who must treat or have contact with patients. Some refuse to treat any HIV patients, for fear of becoming infected themselves and infecting their families. They worry about their careers and the future of their loved ones, should they become infected. Other doctors fear losing some of their clientele if they treat AIDS patients. Still others have a phobia about even the least contact with homosexuals and narcotics addicts. It is not surprising that such cases have been reported in Japan. In Canada and the United States, too, many similar situations have occurred.

BOURGEAULT • Prejudices aside, AIDS patients are victims of discrimination. But I make a distinction between calculated discrimination—from insurance companies, for example, or employers wishing to avoid hiring the wrong kind of people—and discrimination arising more from collective hysteria. In the first case—thanks to charters of human rights, for instance—laws can help, and if not halt, at least curb discriminatory practices in connection with insurance and employment.

IKEDA • Discrimination against patients not only violates medical ethics, but also tramples on human dignity. Surely a sense of human rights must be based on a compassionate, emotionally impartial understanding of others' sufferings.

At an international conference on AIDS held in Vancouver some time ago, a representative of Japanese hemophiliacs spoke of the fact that many Japanese hemophiliacs contracted AIDS from contaminated blood products. AIDS from contaminated blood is currently the number one cause of death among hemophiliacs in Japan. In other words, these people are dying because of the medical products that were supposed to treat their illness.

I believe that the headquarters of the World Hemophiliac Association is in Canada. Have there been similar situations in Canada? What can be done to prevent them?

SIMARD · In retrospect, it is clear that people who need blood transfusions and blood products, like hemophiliacs and patients of major surgery, constitute a group at risk of contamination by blood from an infected donor. Since blood transfusions are easier to control than people's sexual behavior, we could have taken more effective preventative action in dealing with this mode of transmission.

Blood-screening tests have already radically altered the situation. The risk of this kind of transmission in many countries has been practically eliminated by the implementation of very strict public-health measures. Unfortunately, people infected before the development of those blood tests—that is, before 1985—have had, to say the very least, a very painful experience.

IKEDA · We must hope that such a tragedy never repeats itself.

Education and human rights

IKEDA · What methods are now being used in North America to protect the rights of HIV-infected people?

SIMARD · In the United States, it is considered unethical to refuse competent and humane treatment to anyone with AIDS or other conditions related to HIV infection. In Canada, many provinces now prohibit discrimination based on sexual orientation. Quebec and Ontario have passed human-rights legislation prohibiting discrimination based on the perception of a handicap. AIDS will probably qualify as a handicap, so the provincial law will effectively protect patients.

The Royal Society of Canada has recommended that Canadian

human-rights laws be amended specifically to ban discrimination based on evidence of or perception of HIV infection or sexual orientation. Incidentally, many institutions of higher learning, including the University of Montreal, have policies condemning discrimination against HIV carriers and people with AIDS.

IKEDA • A very laudable decision. When a leading institution like the University of Montreal takes action to stop discriminatory practices, it is bound to have a major impact on other medical institutions. Along with official governmental and administrative measures, I think we must also encourage the general public to embrace a view free of discrimination and prejudice, a society that honors human rights.

BOURGEAULT • You are right. As you yourself suggest, we must call for educational activities in the broad sense: widely spreading information, holding events where famous people—actors, for instance—fearlessly demonstrate solidarity and compassion. Every year, in Quebec and all over Canada, large, popular rallies are held—marches in city streets; concerts; shows; and public speeches by politicians, doctors, and so on. Such events help strengthen sympathy for and ties with AIDS patients.

IKEDA • I wish the same level of compassion existed in Japan. Here people are still tested for AIDS surreptitiously—the samples are officially taken for some other purpose—and the results, concealed from the testee, are used in employment policies and school entrance decisions.

BOURGEAULT • Canada has no systematic AIDS screening programs; but tests are made and testees informed of results when, for instance, a blood donation is made. Information campaigns are conducted to encourage target groups to consult specialists and voluntarily submit to testing. Some clinics, like the one in Central-South Montreal, do really remarkable work in this regard.

There are people who would like to have systematic screening put in place for certain groups. Many experts, however, point out that such programs—aside from being likely to encourage stigmatization and discrimination—could represent a double risk to public health. For one thing, people who voluntarily take tests today would henceforth either refuse or at least try to get out of them. For another, screening programs could dull the vigilance of people who don't belong to target groups. Although these programs would be intended to stem the spread of the scourge, they could in fact become its instruments.

IKEDA • As a basic premise, any group testing must respect the human rights of AIDS patients and HIV carriers. Moreover, we must be prudent and circumspect in choosing how to inform patients of their test results. The help of a psychological counselor should be sought and all the issues connected with informed consent should be taken into consideration.

Speaking of human rights reminds me of Dr. John Humphrey (1905–1995), whom I esteem as a great Canadian.

BOURGEAULT • I believe he was one of the authors of the Universal Declaration of Human Rights.

IKEDA • Yes, he was. I met him for the first time in 1993. He not only helped draft the Universal Declaration of Human Rights, but also served for twenty years as the first director of the human rights office at the United Nations Secretariat. I remember that he felt that in building a society dedicated to human rights, education was more important and more effective than legal or organizational coercion.

BOURGEAULT • I imagine he meant human-rights education.

IKEDA • Yes. Now the whole world is calling for organizational human-rights protection to be combined with human-rights education. Dr. Humphrey said that we should make people understand the shame of violating or oppressing others' human rights. We should use education to strengthen public opinion in connection with human rights. Essentially, although the words may sound abstruse, safeguarding human rights actually means protecting human dignity and prizing each human individual, here and now. Buddhists use the term *zanki* which is translated as "humiliation" in this context. The Japanese word means both remorse for one's wrongdoing and shame at one's own misconduct toward others. I believe that developing a sense of *zanki*—a sense of remorse for discrimination and prejudice—is basic to human-rights education.

BOURGEAULT • I think I understand what you are saying, and I agree. I would add to your approach the positive, future-oriented aspect of responsibility. I will come back to that later.

IKEDA • The AIDS problem requires us to hone our sense of the importance of human rights and to combat unacceptable prejudices and false images. The sacred nature of life is more than an abstract concept: it demands that we empathize with sick people and victims of social discrimination and join them in their struggle.

Dr. Lucille Teasdale

BOURGEAULT • That said, I should like, personally, to avoid all reference to the sacred nature of life. Instead, I should like to recall the tremendous admiration generated by the illness and recent death of Lucille Teasdale (1929–96), a Quebecer who, with her husband, built and directed for many years a hospital in Uganda, one of the poorest African nations.

During a complete medical examination in 1985, HIV was detected in her blood. Knowing she was a virus carrier, she mustered her courage and went on with her humanitarian work in Central Africa. She was always on the go, collecting donations for her hospital. In passing, it should be said that she was one of the first women ever to receive an advanced degree from the University of Montreal.

IKEDA • She represents a splendid flowering of the noble educational spirit of your university. Serving others is the kind of human rights struggle that protects human dignity. She risked her life to serve others. Not only the people of Uganda, but all humanity as well will long remember and praise her self-sacrifice.

In one of the sutras, a certain Lady Shrimala makes a sacred vow to Shakyamuni Buddha to protect human rights: "Looking upon them, I cannot forsake the lonely, the unjustly confined and deprived of freedom, sufferers of illness, sufferers of calamity, and the poor. Without fail, I will make their lives tranquil and abundant."

Never forsaking the suffering but risking one's own life to save others—this is true altruism. In Buddhism, we call this the Bodhisattva Way.

BOURGEAULT • Even after contracting AIDS, Lucille Teasdale refused to allow people to pity her fate, remembering the many people around who, in their more painful difficulties, still needed her considerate aid. Until the very end, she was devoted to what she considered her mission.

IKEDA · Through martyrdom to a truly noble cause, she triumphed over the suffering of illness and made a victory of her life.

The AIDS issue is likely to have a seismic effect on religious ethics and the way religions regard morality and sexuality. It is going to stimulate profound reflection on the social mission of religions and what they ought to do for AIDS patients and HIV carriers. The AIDS problem has many facets. HIV infection is deeply related to many such negative aspects of modern civilization as drug abuse, moral and ethical decline, the break-up of the family, and poverty. Religion ought to play a positive role in coping with all of these problems. It must come to head-on grips especially with the spiritual desolation caused by moral and ethical decline and drug addiction.

BOURGEAULT · Religion can and actually does play an ambiguous role. For one thing, the Christian faiths dominant in Canada and Quebec—particularly Roman Catholicism—severely condemn certain sexual practices—homosexuality or extramarital relations, for instance—some of which are not unrelated to the risk of AIDS. Most of them also condemn with equal vehemence the means of avoiding or reducing that risk, particularly condoms. Religious authorities in Quebec have objected to information campaigns in schools and the media promoting condom use.

On the other hand, various groups, some of religious persuasion, others resolutely secular, engage in helping people stricken with AIDS. They have created treatment centers and companion services working either in institutions or in the home. But there is still much to be done. Undeniably, solidarity and compassion are no longer strictly manifested by groups that share the same religious faith. In Quebec and throughout Canada, they transcend former frontiers between religions, as well as between believers and non-believers.

6. Cloning and the Value of Life

Technological feasibility of cloning humans

IKEDA · Now I should like to turn to the topic of cloning.

SIMARD · We can be certain that, in the years to come, cloning is going to be an issue of primary importance to the life sciences.

IKEDA · First, Dr. Simard, just what does *cloning* mean?

SIMARD · The word comes from the Greek *klon* or twig. Briefly, a clone is a group of molecules or cells of the same genetic structure that is descended from one common ancestor. Cloning technology, designed to produce many clones by asexual reproduction—grafting or cuttings, for instance—has proven very useful in animal husbandry, marine biology, and plant and fruit culture.

IKEDA · Given the implications of its application to human beings, how far has cloning advanced? In February 1997, the announcement that the English Dr. Ian Wilmut (1944–) and his colleagues had succeeded for the first time in cloning a sheep from mammary cells obtained from an adult ewe became big news.

SIMARD · Judging from Dr. Wilmut's report on the experiment, I think a human fetus produced by the method he used has a slim chance of developing normally. Dolly, the sheep clone, has now grown up, but no one knows how long she will live[4] or whether she will encounter special problems. We have learned recently that she is fertile, but we do not know what fate awaits her offspring. From a purely scientific standpoint, however, Dr. Wilmut's achievement was a major breakthrough. He and his colleagues claim that it is now technically possible to clone a human being.

IKEDA · But, even if technically possible, is cloning human beings necessary?

SIMARD · Some people assert that a self-clone could be kept as a kind of spare tire to be used at will for organ transplants or other ends.

4. It was recently revealed that Dolly is aging faster than a normal sheep. In fact, her age should eventually become the same as that of the mammary cells of her mother ewe.

Since the organs themselves would be clones, the original organism would not reject them after transplantation. Research into stem cells—embryonic or fetal cells that have preserved their properties of differentiation into various tissues—has a similar goal.

IKEDA • How revolting! This would reduce a human life to nothing more than a bank of spare parts. A mere means to an end.

SIMARD • Exactly. It is the kind of abominable scenario we find in Aldous Huxley's (1894–1963) *Brave New World*.[5] We must not be misled by the title, for the tale Huxley tells is of a hell of human alienation created by mass-producing human clones in a government attempt to establish a perfect social order.

IKEDA • It suggests a nightmarish world devoid of freedom and human rights.

SIMARD • Cloning humans is forbidden in Canada and the United States. Canada does not, however, regulate research on stem cells.

BOURGEAULT • I agree with the principles behind President Clinton and UNESCO's opposition to human cloning.

IKEDA • Article 11 of the Universal Declaration on the Human Genome and Human Rights, adopted by the General Conference of UNESCO (November 11, 1997), states, "Practices which are contrary to human dignity, such as reproductive cloning of human beings, shall not be permitted."

BOURGEAULT • The UNESCO declaration carries great weight because it represents the fruit of intensive discussions among scientists, jurists, and political planners.

Negation of human autonomy and diversity

IKEDA • As a Buddhist, I oppose human cloning as an act that tramples on human dignity. The Buddhist concept of human dignity is grounded on the doctrine of dependent origination (or dependent causation) and the conviction that Buddha nature is inherent in all human beings. The first refers to the interdependence of all phenomena. All beings, including humans, exist or appear through relationships

5. Aldous Huxley. *Brave New World*. London: Chatto and Windus Ed. 1934.

with other beings or phenomena. This means people must live in mutual interdependence and mutual assistance and not seek to satisfy their own desires by sacrificing others. Human cloning treats life as a means to personal benefit. This should be condemned outright.

BOURGEAULT • I agree entirely. Here I refer to the categorical imperative of Immanuel Kant (1724–1804), who has profoundly influenced the tradition of Western thinkers in such matters: an action is morally acceptable only if it is applicable everywhere, with anyone, including oneself. This idea tallies with the golden rule of the ancient Judeo-Christian tradition: "Do unto others as you would have them do unto you."

IKEDA • The idea of self-reflective caring for others is a Buddhist golden rule as well. "Do not give others what you yourself do not want" is a universal ethic throughout Eastern thought, including Buddhism.

BOURGEAULT • If we allow the human being to become a means or instrument to the attainment of some objective—no matter what—we incur the potential danger of reducing all humans to the status of resources.

IKEDA • Human beings are themselves the embodiment of dignity. Human beings must never become mere resources, because this would risk ruining what makes humanity noble. As I mentioned earlier, the Buddhist concept of human dignity also comes from the idea that Buddha nature is inherent in all human beings. Buddha nature, with its infinite potentialities and intrinsic autonomy, manifests itself in diverse forms. The cloning of human beings for reproductive purposes violates human dignity by negating human autonomy and diversity and, by extension, making a mockery of human dignity.

BOURGEAULT • On this point, too, I am in total agreement. Biologically, human beings are created through sexual reproduction, which sets in play a whole gamut of gene combinations. The uniqueness of every individual is a result of this biological process.

In *The Logic of Life*,[6] François Jacob clearly shows how humanity's increasing diversity results from the combination of sexuality and

6. François Jacob. *The Logic of Life: A History of Heredity.* Princeton, New Jersey: Princeton University Press. 1993. See also *The Possible and the Actual.* Seattle: University of Washington Press. 1994.

death: *eros* and *thanatos*. According to him, reproduction by sexual encounter permits the emergence of new living beings and teeming diversity, thanks to the play of genetic combinations. Death makes possible the continuation of that play, of that logic of renewal and diversification.

IKEDA • As you say, Dr. Bourgeault, by stemming diversity, human cloning could suspend or limit human evolution. At the same time, it would raise the question of the nature and meaning of death.

BOURGEAULT • Still, time and again in history, human beings have belied prognoses of catastrophe by surviving apparently insurmountable crises.

IKEDA • I, too, am optimistic about humankind's ability to successfully deal with the technological advances that make human cloning possible. I am convinced that people will resist any impulse to diminish human dignity. The UNESCO declaration is one expression of that wisdom.

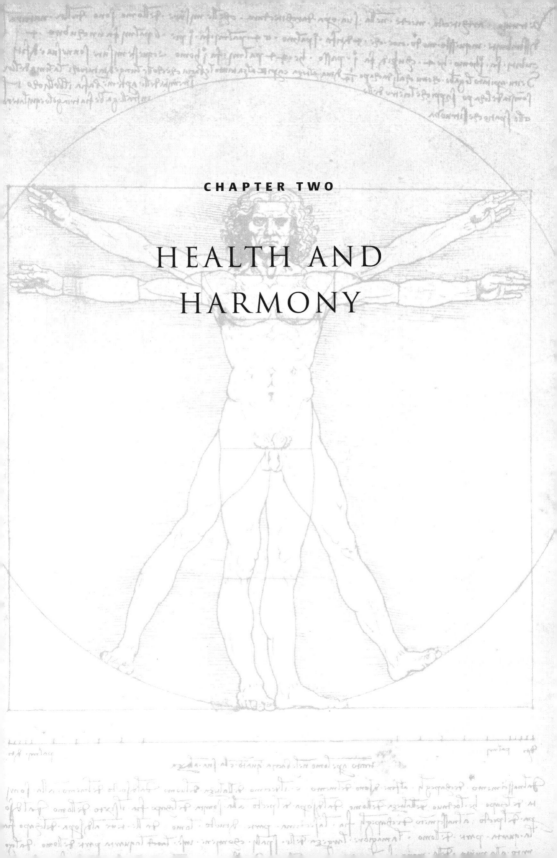

CHAPTER TWO

HEALTH AND HARMONY

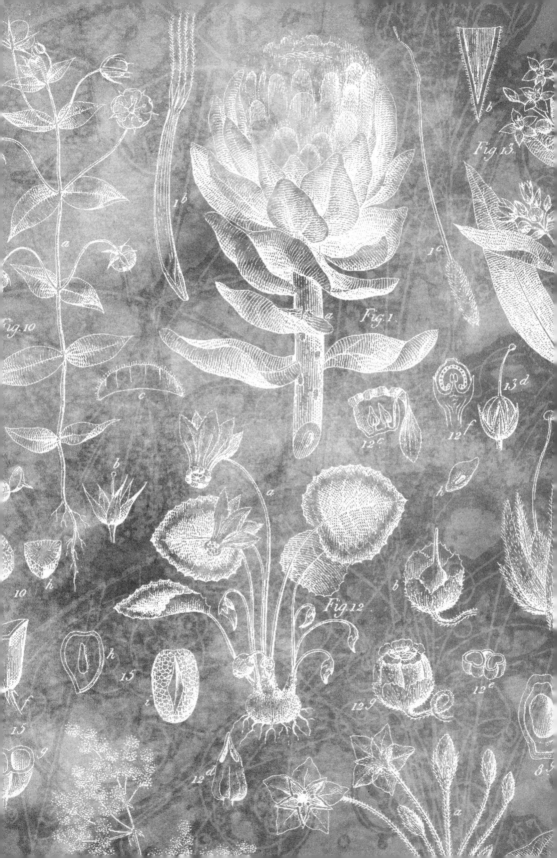

1. The Nature of Health

Dynamic equilibrium

IKEDA • Since Buddhism is a "Law of Life," issues like health and longevity are fundamental to it. Shakyamuni himself gave considerable thought to medical techniques. Buddhist scriptures incorporate the essence of Indian medicine (set forth in the Sacrificial Prayer Veda or *Yajur Veda*), which was the most advanced in the world in its day. At a later stage, Buddhist wisdom on the art of healing was compiled to form what is called Buddhist medicine. The sutras refer to Shakyamuni as the Great Healer. How would you define health, Dr. Bourgeault?

BOURGEAULT • Montaigne (1533–92) once spoke of how much better health seems after an illness.

IKEDA • As everyone knows from experience, we only appreciate how wonderful good health is once we lose it.

BOURGEAULT • In a certain medicine-oriented or simply idealized view, good health is often defined, as you suggest, as the absence of illness or, at least, as the checking or controlling of illness. Just as we breathe without noticing it, we are unaware of health—or of life itself—until it is threatened. Then, all of a sudden, we understand its value.

Immanuel Kant (1724–1804) once observed that we can *feel* well—that is, experience the sensation of vital well-being—but can never know that we *are* well. This is perhaps one of the main reasons medical diagnosis does not always correspond with the experience of the patient. No matter what health may be, defining it is as difficult as giving an adequate definition of life.

IKEDA • Exactly. That is why people sometimes only become aware of their illness once it has advanced until it is beyond treatment. Now please tell me your own view of good health.

BOURGEAULT • Essentially good health is less the absence of illness than the tension between a precarious equilibrium and the constant dynamic of its re-establishment. I like to compare it to walking. Walking is possible only if we are willing to accept the risk of losing our balance by moving forward. A new step temporarily restores the balance until we move still farther forward. A chain of lost and restored balance enables us to walk. A similar process in societies makes history possible.

IKEDA • I like your description of good health as a dynamic rather than static reality. According to the Indian Buddhist sutra The Wanderer's Collection (*Caraka Samhita*), freedom from sickness is fundamental to human life and the basis of good works, success, sexual desire, and liberation from the bonds of illusion and suffering in the three worlds. "Freedom from sickness" means more than the absence of illness. Good health is judged not only on the basis of physiological diagnoses of abnormalities, but also on a holistic view of life that includes spiritual elements.

According to the constitution of the World Health Organization (WHO), health is a state of complete physical, mental, and social well-being, not simply the absence of disease or infirmity. In other words, the concept of good health is not limited to the physical but extends to the spiritual and social as well. How do you feel about the idea of expanding the concept of health to the entirety of human existence?

BOURGEAULT • In one sense, I like the WHO holistic perspective. But this definitely too-ambitious definition of health corresponds to an ideal of vital fullness and integral happiness that is unattainable in reality. It is somewhat naïve to say that health is not only the absence of sickness or infirmity, but also a state of complete physical, mental, and social well-being, no less!

In 1978, the WHO pushed naïveté—rather than audacity—to the point of proposing the goal of "good health for all in 2000." Beyond the slogan, the delusion—and the fantasy—was perfectly obvious.

The definition proposed by Georges Canguilhem (1904–95) in *Britannica Micropaedia* (1992) seems more realistic: Health, in human beings, is the prolonged capacity of an individual to cope physically, emotionally, mentally, and socially with his or her environment. Though similar to the WHO version, this definition makes room for the dynamic of effort and tension I have already mentioned. It reminds us that good health is not a stable state, that it is always threatened, and that we can never take it for granted. Above all, it is never complete and whole, that is, it is never perfect.

IKEDA • Nichiren Daishonin taught that "The four sufferings of birth, old age, sickness and death are the nature of the threefold world."[1] In other words, since all living things must pass through birth, old age, sickness, and death, illness is a natural component of the life cycle. It does not necessarily mean the defeat of life. On the contrary, the struggle to confront illness enables us to celebrate the victory of the human experience. Efforts toward fulfillment are the dynamic of life, and this struggle is the constant equilibrium that you mentioned.

Nichiren Daishonin also said, "Illness gives rise to the resolve to attain the way."[2] Sickness helps people pioneer a more fulfilled way of living by reflecting on the meaning and dignity of life. The very process of overcoming illness tempers body and mind and enables us to create a still broader equilibrium. This is the source of the radiance of good health.

Coping

BOURGEAULT • A friend of mine, stricken with cancer—and now deceased—refused to call himself sick and, above all, to be treated like an invalid. To the very end, he refused to live his life under the sign of sickness and succeeded in "coping"—to borrow Canguilhem's term.

1. *Gosho Zenshu.* 753.
2. *The Writings of Nichiren Daishonin.* Tokyo: Soka Gakkai. 1999. 937.

IKEDA • René Dubos (1901–82), author of *Mirage of Health, Utopias, Progress and Biological Change*,[3] with whom I once conducted a dialogue, considered adaptability to the environment important to good health.

The Buddhist term *myo* (mystic or beyond comprehension) describes a continually creative force that throbs in every healthy entity, sustaining its activities. This force has three general characteristics: renewal, perfection, and openness. The first is a capacity for activation, renewal and creativity. This is demonstrated in the way the human body is constantly called upon to respond in new ways and gather up its creative resources. The second meaning is perfection and completion, in the sense of wholeness and unity. The dynamic equilibrium of the human body as a whole—its homeostatis—bears witness to the action of the mystic force. The third meaning of *myo* is the ideal of openness or the individual's availability to influence his or her environment. Every living thing reacts to its external environment and is capable of provoking a reaction in its environment.

BOURGEAULT • Those three words of the Buddhist tradition—renewal, perfection and openness—are three points of a cyclical continuum, or a helicoid development, in human life. They express what I myself have outlined on several occasions in discussing an evolutionist dynamic of the breakdown and re-establishment of an easily-shattered equilibrium.

Many analysts of change at all levels and on all planes—physical, physiologic and psychological, as well as in relation to social structures and societal evolution—have distinguished between disturbances that occur on the way to establishing a new equilibrium and serious breakdowns. The disturbance in equilibrium seems to be opening the door to chaos, but it is a temporary thing before balance, or equilibrium, is reconstituted into a form hopefully more open than the one that went before. No doubt I am sacrificing a few of the nuances in comparing this to the Buddhist viewpoint you describe— but perhaps, when all is said and done, not entirely.

---

3. René Dubos. *Mirage of Health, Utopias, Progress and Biological Change.* New Jersey: Rutgers University Press. 1987.

IKEDA • What can you tell me about the genetic interpretation of health and illness?

BOURGEAULT • One might say that genetics today "internalizes" illness, and health along with it. It claims that, at the heart of what makes a person an individual living being, a defect, error, or genetic flaw—or at least a predisposition or risk—causes internal imbalance or an incapacity to interrelate adequately with the environment.

Indirectly, these definitions refer back to a "normality," a rectitude, and a perfection, and therefore an implicit norm never defined and undoubtedly indefinable. This is a statistical normality that relates to no real individual. It is an ideal and totally unreal normality. But of course, any kind of "normality"—even if we are not aware of it—establishes a norm.

IKEDA • I am afraid that such an ambiguous standard of normality could promote discrimination.

BOURGEAULT • Yes, there is that risk, notably in drafting health policies. A few years ago, at the Research Center on Public Law at the University of Montreal, I headed a team that was working on the role of ideas of anomaly, handicap, and genetic illnesses in the development and management of health-related policies in Quebec and across Canada.

The development of genetic medicine and epidemiology as instruments of public prevention policy runs the risk of being accompanied by a certain stigmatization of targeted populations. Discriminatory behavior is imputable to inadequate understanding of genetics and to equating the illness with the gene and the gene with the person.

A deeper understanding of health and illness, handicap and incapacity, anomaly and abnormality, and the full gamut of intermediary stages is of crucial importance.

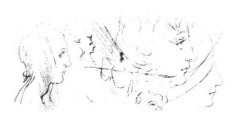

2. Health and Illness

The oneness of sickness and health

IKEDA • Have you ever been ill?

BOURGEAULT • Not really. I have experienced illness only indirectly—if I can put it that way—through the sickness that struck my older brother—now deceased—when I was a child and later when some of my friends became seriously sick. I had a high fever when I was four, but it went down fairly fast. A few days later, it struck my nine-year-old brother, who then suffered from polio and its after-effects until his death at fifty-five.

IKEDA • At that time, the polio vaccine was not yet available. So you really experienced the suffering of illness through your brother.

BOURGEAULT • At first I felt guilty. Later, perhaps I simply became very attentive to sick people because I enjoyed the privilege of good health.

IKEDA • What you just said reminds me of the story of the Mahayana bodhisattva Vimalakirti who, though actually in good health, pretends to be ill out of empathy with sick and suffering sentient beings. In the story told in the *Vimalakirti Sutra*, Shakyamuni suggests that his disciples pay a sick call on him. But Shariputra, Ananda, and the other Disciples of Learning are reluctant to go and see him. Finally, Monjushiri, one of the most outstanding of the bodhisattvas, visits Vimalakirti's sickroom, along with some other bodhisattvas and Disciples of Learning and Realization. When Monjushiri asks, "What is your illness?" Vimalakirti answers, "I am ill because other beings are ill. When they are healed, I too will be healed."

The message is that the bodhisattva's illness is the result of his great compassion and his sense of responsibility for the sufferings of all other beings. Your own sense of responsibility toward those who are suffering from illness is very similar to the idea of Buddhist compassion. Buddhism teaches that good health and sickness are one and inseparable. This unifying vision of health illustrates the links that tie each individual to the suffering of others, creating a radiant picture of human health.

BOURGEAULT · I like your way of understanding good health and sickness as inseparable. The relationship between health and illness—the latter being a revealing reflection of the former—is complex. There is more than simple opposition between the obverse and reverse—between health and illness.

IKEDA · Modern molecular biology and biotechnology are making astonishing progress. New substances are being created and new ways of synthesizing natural substances are being discovered. Many of them are producing impressive results in disease treatment. One of the fascinating aspects of these recent developments is the discovery that the human body was designed to naturally produce substances such as insulin and morphine. In other words, an organism in "good working order" is able to produce these natural "drugs" in sufficient quantities.

BOURGEAULT · The natural forces of the cosmos and of living beings are indeed extraordinary. I am always dazzled by the amazing capacity of the living being to restore life in spite of obstacles or breakdowns. This capacity is miraculous in the etymological sense of the word. But the play of natural forces is not always without catastrophe. I am thinking about the kinds of things that high-flown sermons on the "return to Nature" overlook: volcanic eruptions, typhoons, tidal waves, and the totally natural disappearance of certain species.

IKEDA · True. Life does have negative aspects, at least on the surface.

BOURGEAULT · While the human organism possesses remarkable forces of healing or restoration of internal equilibrium and health—even of regeneration—it also has destructive elements, such as over- or underproduction of insulin and renal dysfunction necessitating regular dialysis to ward off poisoning and death. While we can be confident in the natural forces of the organism, we must also know how to compensate for their insufficiencies and sometimes modify the rules of the game in order to correct unfortunate trajectories.

IKEDA · Yes. Too much insulin produces harmful side effects. Too little hinders the health of the organism. A hyperactive immune system, rather than protecting the body from outside enemies, can result in so-called autoimmune illnesses like Basedow's disease (exophthalmic goitre), *myasthenia gravis*, and other recalcitrant conditions.

It is true that we know little about this, or about the way the body functions. We cannot define superfluity and insufficiency in simple terms, so we must take a multifaceted view of life itself. In addition, we must further explore the "rules" that regulate the body's inherent healing powers.

BOURGEAULT · We must guard against blind faith in nature—specifically the natural self-healing capacity of the human organism—and take into consideration the risks of using medication (in the strict sense of pharmaceutical products). The use of medication grows at a startling rate. We now know that while certain treatments and medications enable us to save lives or improve the condition and quality of life, they may have harmful side effects. For example, the role of antibiotics is to combat bacterial infection. They can also, however, weaken and even upset the functioning of the immune system.

Generally, simple responses and solutions are illusory. We would like to be able to say that whatever is "natural" is for that reason good. Similarly we would like to be able to say that whatever is artificial—the product of artifice (art and science)—if not always bad, inevitably induces risk because it changes the rules of the game by modifying the natural course of things. But actually the natural course of things sometimes leads to catastrophe if artifice does not divert it in the desired direction.

The teeming complexity of interactions occurring constantly "inside" the human organism and with the very numerous forces of the exterior environment condemns all interventions in the biomedical field to ambivalence and ambiguity. These interventions, which simultaneously make and unmake the order of things, cannot eliminate one risk without introducing another.

We can nevertheless greet as promising research and therapy that aim to instate a new equilibrium and new relations between "nature" and "artifice." As one example among many, it is now possible to produce insulin outside the body for later injection when the rhythm of internal insulin production is insufficient. This provides new impetus to what you have called the body's pharmaceutical factory. But who knows how far we will be able to go on that impetus.

A new genetic therapy has recently enabled Robert Tanguay, of Laval University, and Marcus Grompe, of the Oregon University of

Sciences and Health, to reconstruct complete livers inside living mice, using a few genetically modified cells. No doubt, genetic therapy, in which artifice helps nature, will soon be called upon to play an important role in stimulating the forces of internal regeneration in human beings.

Recipes for health

IKEDA • I'd like to ask you a few questions about nutrition. Is there a particular type of food that can invigorate the mind? Linus Pauling (1901–94), the father of modern chemistry and a celebrated researcher on vitamin C, looked perplexed when I asked him that question. I don't expect a definitive scientific answer. I'm simply curious about your opinion.

BOURGEAULT • My wife is a dietician, but that does not make me an expert in the field. I only know, for example, that children who do not eat breakfast find it hard to pay attention in class. That is why, for almost twenty years, breakfasts have been served every morning in schools in the so-called underprivileged parts of Montreal.

IKEDA • In his book *The Education of Man*, Friedrich Froebel (1782–1852) says that, depending on whether or not children eat breakfast, they will be industrious or lazy, lively or indecisive, quick or dull-witted, energetic or listless. In Japan today, the number of children who do not or cannot eat breakfast is said to be growing.

BOURGEAULT • We know that malnutrition—or what the specialists call "undernutrition"—can irreparably damage the brain. But I know of no work that has established an irrefutable link between any particular food and intellectual vigor.

IKEDA • I suppose we will have to wait for corroborative research in brain sciences and nutrition. Do you yourself follow any specific health regimens?

BOURGEAULT • I have never gone in for sports. In high school and college I always had my nose in a book. A teacher once told me I was jeopardizing my health and that I would not last long, but I have now rounded the sixty mark—possibly out of sheer belligerence. When I was little, my mother used to say that if I ever fell into a river, she would send the lifeguards to fish me out upstream instead of downstream. I do, however, observe two principles for staying in good health.

IKEDA • Tell us what they are.

BOURGEAULT • One is to free my mind when I have finished a task of, for instance, writing or teaching, even when I know that I could have gone farther and done better. The other is walking on an almost daily basis. But, most important of all, I think I have inherited what we call "good genes."

3. Harmony with the Environment

Six causes of illness

IKEDA • The great Chinese Buddhist teacher T'ien-t'ai (538–597) posits six causes of sickness that cover problems arising from dietary habits, viral infections—such as polio—mental disorders and genetic heritage.

First, sickness results from disharmony among the four elements—earth, water, fire, and wind—that make up the human body and correspond to the physical states solid, liquid, thermal and gaseous. This disharmony can result from an inability to adapt to changes in the external environment—weather, for example. Second come illnesses arising from poor dietary habits or irregular mealtimes. Third are sicknesses said to be caused by irregular meditation. In other words, when there are disturbances in the rhythm of our lives—such as insufficient sleep and exercise—we are susceptible to illness.

The fourth cause of illness T'ien-t'ai mentions is quite interesting: "news from a demon." In modern terms, this demon could be something like bacteria or viruses or external psychological stress. The fifth cause is the influence of malevolent forces. The chaotic instincts and desires inherent in human nature unbalance the functions of the body and the mind. Buddhism teaches that mental illnesses arise mainly from delusions like wrath and greed. Sixth are karma-caused sicknesses. Buddhism and other Indian religions teach that life transmigrates from the past, to the present, and into the future because of the powerful energy of karma, which may be called potential life energy. Consequently, physical and psychological genetic makeup reflects past karma. According to the distinctively Buddhist interpretation, distortions in that energy can cause sickness.

The oneness of life and its environment

IKEDA • Let us further discuss the relationship between the human body and the environment—or what T'ien-t'ai calls disharmony among the four elements. In speaking of the environment and human life, Nichiren Daishonin said, "The ten directions are the 'environment,' and living beings are 'life.' Environment is like the shadow, and life, the body. Without the body, no shadow can exist, and without life, no environment. In the same way, life is shaped by its environment."[4] In other words, at the fundamental level, the environment and the living body are one and mutually influence each other. Buddhism refers to this doctrine as the oneness of life and its environment.

BOURGEAULT • I see.

IKEDA • During the long process of evolution, the human body repeatedly adapted to the external environment by acquiring a capacity to regulate the internal environment. In our modern scientific civilization, however, where environmental pollution and destruction present serious challenges, we confront material circumstances for which we have no adaptive mechanisms. If we do not now follow the Buddhist teaching of the oneness of life and its environment and learn to live in harmony and peaceful coexistence with the global ecology, we will put not only ourselves, but also every other living thing on Earth in jeopardy.

In times like these, what must we do to maintain dynamic harmony with the global environment and enable humanity to enjoy a healthy way of life?

BOURGEAULT • Today, the preservation and restoration of the environment are a question of life and death, of health or illness, for us and for our children and grandchildren.

4. *The Writings of Nichiren Daishonin.* 644.

In a sense, the history of human intervention in the environment goes back as far as humanity itself. Technological and industrial developments of the last decades, however, have fantastically widened the field for human environmental intervention. That is the novelty. A qualitative breakdown—made up of many fragmentations—has taken place. This is what makes ethical judgment crucially important. Should human beings do what we are able to do simply because we can? Is it appropriate? Is it advantageous? And, if so, advantageous to whom?

In these affairs I reject both wide-eyed optimism and anguished pessimism. To my mind, active lucidity opens a middle way between naïveté and cynicism.

A sense of responsibility demanded by scientific and technological development

IKEDA • The release of nuclear energy took technoscientific progress to an extreme. Even peaceful uses of nuclear power cause serious environmental pollution. The disastrous Chernobyl accident in 1986 was by far the worst environmental disaster to date. The immediate effects of the deadly radioactive fallout were terrible, but it was only afterward, when radioactive contamination was found in neighboring countries, that people fully grasped the extent of the damage to water and the food chain.

The possibility of environmental pollution from the large-scale nuclear power plants and nuclear-energy facilities being built all over the world stimulates debate and arouses a sense of crisis on national and global levels. Government authorities and experts urge the public to avoid unfounded fears and trust reasonable judgments, but this did not prevent the Chernobyl disaster and the extensive spread of deadly pollution despite all efforts to minimize the tragedy.

BOURGEAULT • The abundance of hydroelectric resources in Canada explains why we have built only a few nuclear power plants. But they, too, have had their "little failures." Canada has exported its nuclear technology—the Candu—to a number of countries, notably India.

Personally, I react with distrust to what both ardent defenders and detractors of nuclear energy have to say. The former solemnly affirm the great security of nuclear facilities and cite control measures and systems so rigorous that risks are minimal—in theory, zero. The latter periodically cite the incidence—and extent—of startling genetic malformations and diverse illnesses in regions contaminated without the knowledge of local inhabitants. Once again, I refuse to be forced to choose either unconditional trust or suspicious vigilance.

IKEDA • In the late 1990s, accidents involving radioactive leakage occurred at several of the facilities operated by the Japanese Power Reactor and Nuclear Fuel Development Corporation. Worse yet, the company tried to conceal them and presented falsified reports to the government authorities. This unforgivable irresponsibility stirred up considerable distrust and criticism from all quarters. If there is a lesson to be learned from these accidents, it is that responsibility for operating nuclear energy facilities must be made clear, and entire operations must be open to scrutiny.

BOURGEAULT • Even when the equally undeniable advantages and risks are taken into consideration, recourse to nuclear energy, in whatever form and to whatever end, should not be envisioned without rigorous supervision.

IKEDA • I agree completely.

BOURGEAULT • To act in a responsible manner is to recognize risk and, if it cannot be entirely eliminated, appropriate measures should be taken to reduce its impact. We still have not found a place where nuclear waste can be stockpiled with complete safety for the coming centuries.

IKEDA • A keen sense of responsibility is extremely important in all environmental issues.

BOURGEAULT • Absolutely. Another important aspect of an ethic of responsibility concerns intergenerational relationships.

IKEDA • We must not continue to destroy the environment for the sake of present generations when this means inflicting suffering on future generations. In addition to intergenerational problems, we face interregional conflicts as well. For instance, opposition between the North and South greatly impeded efforts for environmental conservation at the United Nations Conference on Environment and Development held in Brazil in 1992.

BOURGEAULT · The situation is all the graver because nuclear plants are not the only menace to environmental quality. In recent years we have become increasingly aware of the destructive nature of a certain mode of industrial and technological development. Instead of renouncing or changing methods of production and technologies that do not conform to the strict norms of the countries in the North, large international enterprises export them to countries in the South—in the guise of regional development! This is being done under the banner of the noble cause of economic globalization and business restructuring. Even non-recyclable production wastes from northern countries are exported to poor nations, as is sometimes revealed when the media follow maritime cargoes from port to port and on to their eventual destination. No doubt, however, many "deliveries" of such "merchandise" escape their vigilance.

IKEDA · Tropical rainforests in such timber-exporting Southeast-Asian countries as the Philippines, Thailand, and Malaysia are being destroyed. One of the causes is excessive felling in response to the Japanese liberalization of lumber imports in the 1960s.

Pollution today does not remain within national borders but spreads to every part of the world. Destruction of the Arctic ozone layer—on Canada's threshold—is connected with global increases in ultraviolet rays that damage human beings, animals and crops. Many nations are co-operating to control the production of devices that emit chlorofluorocarbons, which deplete the ozone layer, but it is clear that the policies and countermeasures of a few countries acting independently are no longer enough to solve the world-scale problem of our times.

BOURGEAULT · You are quite right. The deterioration of the ozone layer is causing increasing anxiety in Canada. Awareness of this matter increases proportionally with fear in the face of mounting skin-cancer rates. We are equally disturbed by global warming and its consequences. But, for all that, behavior remains unchanged—or changes very little.

IKEDA · Canada is world-famous for the beautiful lakes and vast forests of its wonderful natural environment. What role and mission do you see for your country in dealing with global-problem syndromes?

BOURGEAULT · The work and recommendations of the Brundtland Commission, the publication of reports in the media, symposia and conferences—like the meeting in Montreal some years ago—have aroused unprecedented awareness of the deterioration of the environment and of the possibility of redressing the situation—at a price. A public opinion poll conducted in 1989 put environmental issues in first place among the concerns of the Canadian people. A poll conducted in the United States in 1990 showed that 74% of the population felt that, even if they are costly, necessary steps to preserve and improve the quality of the environment must not be further postponed. Ten years later, however, rising unemployment seems to have put economic issues—what are sometimes called economic "imperatives"—back in first place.

An environmental ethics of sustainable development

IKEDA · In Japan, too, awareness of environmental issues is increasing little by little. People are especially concerned about the harmful effects of the chemical byproducts of incinerators. One survey showed that 80% of the population is familiar with the term "environmental hormones."

The public debate brought about by the 1997 Kyoto Agreement on climatic changes and greenhouse gases helped make the Japanese people more aware of such global issues as the restriction of carbon dioxide emissions. Extensive media coverage of the meeting certainly had a great impact on the public.

UN officials and other people concerned with environmental issues frequently repeat the mantra of "sustainable development."

BOURGEAULT · In 1987, the World Commission on Environment and Development, presided over by Mrs. Gro Harlem Brundtland (1939–), presented the General Assembly of the United Nations with a report very significantly entitled *Our Common Future*.[5] Attempting to reconcile the proponents of development (principally, if not exclusively, economic) and those of the protection and preservation

5. World Commission on Environment and Development (UN). *Our Common Future*. Oxford: Oxford University Press. 1987.

of the environment, the report proposed as a compromise a course of integration and an inclusive perspective referred to as sustainable development.

There was nothing radically new in the proposal, which restates, fifteen years later, the manifesto of the Stockholm Conference devoted to humanity in its environment: *Only One Earth*.[6] The resources of our small planet are not unlimited. As has already been said, we must use them with prudence and foresight, in a way that does not exhaust them but ensures their constant renewal.

Nonetheless, it fell to the Brundtland Commission to give new impetus to the dissemination of these ideas, this perspective, and this course of action. Its members called for solidarity, justice, and especially the need for equity between present and future generations. They showed that the proposed change in direction is feasible if we resolutely undertake to devote to sustainable development the sums now invested in armament (more than US$1000 billion a year).

According to the Brundtland Commission, humanity has no future unless we reconcile the demands of development with protection of the quality of the environment in a dynamic of sustainable development. Among other preliminary conditions, this dynamic requires peace, justice, respect for the rights of everyone, and solidarity between nations and generations.

IKEDA • I picture environmental ethics as an axis around which reform within individual human beings that will make sustainable development possible will revolve.

First, the premise of environmental ethics must be the practice of non-violence and peace arising from the concept of the dignity of life. Efforts to create a non-violent world will enable us to redirect the vast sums now spent on war and armaments to environmental conservation.

Second, since the environment is necessarily limited, we require an ethics that allows us to live within those limitations. We must convert the greed-driven, extravagant lifestyle of the industrialized nations into a lifestyle in which we control our desires. Third, our ethics

6. Barbara Ward and René Dubos. *Only One Earth: The Care and Maintenance of a Small Planet*. New York: W.W. Norton. 1972.

must be based on a vision that will inspire and help not only the people of today, but also future generations. Consider the way we manage our economies: unless we can make a transition to a cyclical concept in which constant economic growth is not a "given," we will compromise the environment for future generations.

BOURGEAULT • An ethic for sustainable development demands profound changes in mentality and behavior. We must learn to think in terms of systems instead of the compartments we are accustomed to. We must act in solidarity, all the while respecting differentiation of the responsibilities and tasks of various partners.

IKEDA • We of the SGI seek to create solidarity from a global perspective with everybody, no matter how much their standpoints differ from our own.

BOURGEAULT • Admittedly, until the present, thinking in compartments has permitted the development of scientific knowledge. Now, however, to proceed further, science must take into consideration the interactions within a complex play of interdependencies. In addition, we must learn a sense of moderation—moderation imposed both by the limits of our resources and ecological requirements and by justice. We must learn friendliness and cooperation among ourselves, beyond our borders, and also between ourselves and other living beings and the natural environment. We must learn shared responsibility, with a view to collective action and synergy.

IKEDA • The fourth environmental ethic derives from the idea of coexistence. Its major element is recognition of the right to life not only of humans, but also of animals and all other living things. To internalize the philosophy of harmonious human coexistence with the environment, we need to actively promote environmental education.

BOURGEAULT • Like you, I believe that only education can help us develop a responsible ethic permitting us to confront the issues of today and tomorrow. In the medium and long term, the route to regulating technological development must be through ethics and education.

4. Obsession with Perpetual Youth

The quest for eternity and a meaningful present

BOURGEAULT · The so-called Western nations have long been influenced by Judeo-Grecian-Christian thought. People shared a hope of and belief in life after death. Today, in their uncertainty about post-mortem life, they prefer to give meaning to their existences by living as fully as possible now.

IKEDA · Although living *now* with all our might is important, if we lose sight of the idea that the present exists for the future, we run the risk of lapsing into Epicureanism.

BOURGEAULT · Life has in store for everyone so many annoyances and such misery that it would be difficult to give oneself up to the blessed satisfaction of the pleasure of the moment. It is true, however, that there exists, especially in the countries of North America and Europe, a certain cult of happiness—a duty to be happy, even a right to happiness. I refer to this as the Japanese-car syndrome.

As you know, for twenty years now, many of the cars on the streets of Quebec have been of Japanese make. The increase in the number of these vehicles is partly the result of a policy of full guarantee on parts and labor provided by the Japanese manufacturers. The "bumper-to-bumper guarantee" means that in case of breakdown, defect or even sometimes accident, the purchaser is entitled to repairs free of charge, or even to a new car. Sometimes, we interpret our relationship with our bodies, our health and our quality of life in a similar way. In other words, misfortune simply has to be the result of faulty manufacture. Therefore the responsibility rests with the Creator, the parents, or the delivering doctor. And we demand repairs or, at least, compensation.

IKEDA · It is a clever metaphor. According to Buddhist teachings, some sicknesses and disabilities are attributed to karma, as I said earlier. This means that we must delve deeply into life itself to understand certain physical or mental conditions.

In monotheistic religions, God is called the "Creator." It is he who made human beings and everything that exists in the universe. But some people are born with congenital or hereditary malformations, and others with disabilities. There is a host of possible answers, not all of them convincing, to the question of why God created evil.

As you say, people today think above all of getting the most out of life, of living in a way that makes sense of life. But it seems to me that behind this need to make sense out of life, there lies a propensity for the eternal. If life were nothing but present existence, theoretically Epicureanism would be perfectly acceptable. But most people want to follow the path of good. The very idea of wanting to live righteously indicates intuitive awareness of something eternal.

BOURGEAULT · On this point our views differ. Eternal life seems to me to be a desire, a dream, but not a reality. Mere wishful thinking. Desire does not create reality. Like Jean-Paul Sartre (1905–80), I believe we can live in compassion and solidarity and give our existence the meaning we desire, even if there is no life after death—no life after this one. Giving meaning to life is simultaneously an issue of human liberty and a challenge, a responsibility.

IKEDA · It is only natural that our views should differ on some issues. The Buddhist scripture called *Majjima-nikaya* (The Middle-Length Sayings) contains a passage saying, "Do not chase after the past, do not long for the future . . . Who knows? Death may come tomorrow. Just do in earnest what must be done today." Though its basic view of life and death differs from Sartre's, it shares with him the idea of living enthusiastically in the single moment we call *now*, in the single day we call *today* and in this life. On this specific point perhaps we agree, you and I.

BOURGEAULT · The universe was here long before me and will remain when I am gone. We are made of the same matter as the stars. To repeat the lovely title of Hubert Reeves's book, we are "stardust."[7] Our life is only a piece, a fragment, of an immensely more inclusive life.

IKEDA · You speak of human life as part of a much more inclusive life. Similarly, Buddhism teaches that we human beings contain within ourselves the great entity of cosmic life. Not only are our bodies

7. Hubert Reeves. *Poussières d'étoiles*. Paris: Éditions du Seuil, coll. "Science ouverte." 1984.

made of the same matter as the universe, but our minds are also united with the cosmos at a deep level. This principle is known as "three thousand realms in a single life-moment (*ichinen-sanzen*)." Our life is the single life-moment, and the three thousand realms are cosmic life. Both spiritually and physically, our life is one with the universe; in other words, the self equals the cosmos.

BOURGEAULT • Someone once said that astonishment was the origin of philosophy—and of poetry, too, no doubt. I recall contemplating the starry sky when I was an adolescent. I still do it today. Nonetheless, I am convinced that I have only this life to live, my own, limited yet so precious.

IKEDA • That is true. Precious and irreplaceable.

Transforming the four sufferings into elation and happiness

IKEDA • By the way, according to the Buddhist view, we can live to be 120, as Nichiren makes clear in the following passage: "It is better to live a single day with honor than to live to 120 and die in disgrace."[8] What do you think is the maximum age to which we can live?

BOURGEAULT • Some say that, given optimal conditions, we can really attain the respectable age of 120, or even more. Others maintain that age limit is registered in each person's genetic clock. I discovered my own mortality when I reached the age of fifty—late in life, my friends tell me. In spite of my resolute optimism, I found myself compelled to embark on the downhill side of my life.

IKEDA • In the aging societies of industrialized nations like Japan and Canada, everyone must directly face the questions of both how to live and how to die with dignity. Medical science has studied the human aging phenomenon from various angles. Some say life span is determined by the limits of cell division. Others claim that aging is genetically controlled. What are your opinions on the aging process?

BOURGEAULT • Undoubtedly the secret desire for eternal youth has nourished many dreams. Certain fairy tales that have become classics of Western literature bear me out in this. I am sure the same is true in

8. *The Writings of Nichiren Daishonin.* 851.

Japan as well. Developments in biomedical science and technology have undoubtedly revived dormant desires for eternal youth. So far we have managed to prolong life without being able to restore to it the vigor of youth. As the great French diet and nutrition specialist Jean Trémolières was fond of saying, the important thing is not to add years to life but to add life to years.

My personal attitudes toward aging—and more indirectly toward death—are stamped with ambivalence. Surely I am not alone in this. There is no Golden Age. There are no Good Old Times. In his novel *Write to Kill: A Sentimental Journey from the Source to the Black Sea,* novelist and teacher Daniel Pennac (1944–) has the protagonist, Malaussène, say: "At whatever age, life is an utter bitch: childhood, the age of tonsils and total dependence; adolescence, the age of onanism and pointless questioning; maturity, the age of cancer and rampant bullshit; old age, the age of arthritis and vain regret."[9]

IKEDA • Such biting satire! But it is also poignant, because it describes the four sufferings of birth, aging, sickness, and death.

BOURGEAULT • Pennac's iconoclastic and deliberately offensive and provocative comments seem somehow related to the Buddhist tradition of the four sufferings. The difficulty of living tinges all stages of existence.

IKEDA • Yes, as you suggest, Buddhism interprets the hard realities of life as the four sufferings, which are innate and inherent in life itself for all human beings.

In addition to these four general categories, Buddhism examines more specific sufferings as well. First is the necessity of parting from our loved ones. For various reasons, we must all part with people we love, and these partings are all sad, no matter how much we love the people we're obliged to leave. The ultimate form of separation is, of course, death. Second is the necessity of encountering people we hate. Experiencing resentment and animosity, at home or at work, is demoralizing. Third is the impossibility of attaining what we desire— whether our desire is spiritual, psychological, material, or social. In industrialized countries, people may be satisfied in material and social

9. Daniel Pennac. *Write to Kill: A Sentimental Journey from the Source to the Black Sea.* Tr. Ian Monk. London: Harvill Press. 1999. 100.

terms, but many still experience profound frustration on the spiritual and existential planes, a frustration centered on the question of how they can live a fulfilling life. Feelings of general powerlessness, pessimism and depression are the symptoms of being unable to answer this question.

These seven kinds of suffering are considered inevitable as long as the "five components" of life—form, perception, conception, volition and consciousness—are active. These components are the foundation for all life operations, physical and mental. As long as we remain alive, our bodies are active and our minds are constantly changing. The suffering that arises from these activities is inherent in life. Starting from these hard realities, Buddhism shows how suffering can be transformed into true joy, not simply physical pleasure.

BOURGEAULT · We fool ourselves with illusions of laughing childhood, gilded youth, the assured success of mature age, and the wisdom of the old. Perhaps we actually recognize them to be delusions. There is no *best* time in life, perhaps for the sound reason that all times in life can be good. There are no givens: nothing is either assured or irreparably lost.

IKEDA · A French writer once compared life to the flow of a river: youth is like a torrent, maturity a rapid river, and old age a great waterway reflecting the surrounding scenery like a mirror and finally emptying into the ocean.

Each person experiences the transition from childhood, to adolescence, to young adulthood, maturity, and finally old age. In youth, torrent-like, we live headlong. In maturity, we face the growing responsibilities of family and society. Next comes a period of deep reflection on the meaning of life—a time of wisdom and completion. Then comes the final summing up as, from the standpoint of old age, we look into the face of death.

An open, pliable and tolerant mind

BOURGEAULT · As I have already said, ambivalence colors my attitudes toward aging. Increasing age means often slow, enriching maturation, accompanied by an irremediable decline in energy. Ours is a strange situation: we must consent to lose in order to gain.

IKEDA • You are right. We gain experience as we pass through the various stages of life. The depth, breadth, and confidence of the views of life and death we evolve in the process determine whether we triumph or fail. In this sense, we all hope that growing old will mean growing as a human being, that it will be a process that leads us to our full potential as individuals.

BOURGEAULT • In the past, I often told people that I felt younger at 30 than I had at 20 and younger at 40 than I had at 30. Beyond the fifty-year mark, I stopped saying this. Had I really been talking of youth? Sifting through my memories, I seemed to be more at my ease. I was "in better possession of my resources," as people sometimes say. More experienced. More secure and for that reason more open and ready for new encounters, new friendships, and new challenges.

IKEDA • Your splendid process of self-actualization reveals how, while overcoming the four sufferings, you expanded your environment to the scale of a great ocean. You have experienced the ideal life.

BOURGEAULT • Not at all. As I said, at 50, I hesitated to say that I felt younger than I had at 40. I wondered whether I wasn't deluding myself to claim I was staying young. I began to feel strongly that I ought to be responsible for and to young people (those of my own family and the students I met and worked with) for the future life they would live when I was no longer among them.

IKEDA • The real meaning of youth has nothing to do with physical age. In Buddhist terms, youth means the open-mindedness—pliability and tolerance—of the life-moment (*ichinen*).

BOURGEAULT • I consider it mistaken to associate openness and flexibility with youth and obtuse rigidity with old age. In practical experience—which, of course, varies from one person to another—things are much more nuanced.

IKEDA • Very true. Many older people are enthusiastically active in society, do creative work, or perform social services. They demonstrate acute powers of observation and broad judgment based on a rich store of experience, and they continue to study and to learn. They constantly absorb new knowledge and have minds that are truly open to society and life. For these people, old age is akin to writing the final chapter of their lives, the purpose of which is to perfect themselves as individuals. Their lives are founded on creativity, hope, and joy.

BOURGEAULT · It seemed easier for me to be open and to accept new things when I was 40 and even 50 than it had been when I was 20.

IKEDA · One of the Buddhist scriptures reads, "You will grow younger, and your good fortune will accumulate."[10]

The importance of new encounters

BOURGEAULT · At 50, I had to give in to the evidence that I would be unable to visit all the countries on earth, let alone the planets and stars of the innumerable galaxies of the universe.

IKEDA · I have circled the globe several times and visited many countries, but there are still so many that I haven't visited.

BOURGEAULT · I shall die without discovering cities rich in history and culture, without meeting and exchanging ideas with many people— both men and women—with whom I share a common humanity transcending boundaries traced in space and time, and without having read so many of the books I want to read. For a while this thought made me profoundly sad. But the sadness dissipated quickly.

IKEDA · Did something happen to cause this change?

BOURGEAULT · Instead of pursuing the new and unknown, I went—for perhaps the thirtieth time—to Paris, where I love to stroll aimlessly in the streets and parks. I suddenly saw that what I needed was to live more fully and to savor what had been given me to know. I realized that I needed to overcome, from within, limitations that seemed to have been stifling me. After the breathlessness of the race, I needed to find the rhythm of slow, deep breathing.

Then all of a sudden I was 60, without trying or even thinking about it. Then I felt even more keenly a desire to exchange ideas with people younger than me. My aim was not only to teach them what I knew, but also to learn from them and, perhaps, to avoid growing old too fast. I wanted to prevent my sensibilities from dulling too rapidly by stimulating them through associations with newer sensibilities. It

10. *The Writings of Nichiren Daishonin.* 464.

is impossible to teach for more than 40 years and not be profoundly affected by it! I saw that we learn by teaching and that we can teach passionately and communicate the pleasure of learning only if we preserve our own thirst for learning. It seems to me that societies and individuals need to establish new relationships between generations.

IKEDA • That is exactly what the famous exhortation "know thyself" means. You not only reoriented yourself, you discovered your true self.

The goal of Buddhism is also self-knowledge. To know his true self, Shakyamuni abandoned his royal position, rejected earthly pleasures, and endured terrible privations. He went on to reject asceticism and advocate a way of life that transcends the extremes of self-indulgence and self-denial. Savoring the rhythm of the Middle Way, he became enlightened and discovered his cosmic self, which we call the Buddha. And this was the start of Shakyamuni Buddha's mission to save all sentient beings.

BOURGEAULT • Love, friendship, and meeting people have become more important for me than ever. I appreciate the privilege of teaching more.

IKEDA • Shakyamuni is sometimes called the Teacher of Humanity. In Buddhist thought, compassion is a process of eliminating suffering and giving happiness. It suggests sharing the four sufferings, triumphing over them and winning true happiness. Originally the term *compassion* connoted friendship. Compassion, friendship, and encounters with other people are symbols of youth. They are the rewards of lifelong youthfulness.

5. Overcoming Stress

Mother and daughter: sharing the battle against cancer

BOURGEAULT • In your discussion with Dr. Simard you asked whether it is desirable to inform patients that they have cancer. If you don't mind, I would like to add my "two cents' worth."

IKEDA • Please, by all means. It would be a shame to miss out on what an authority on bioethics has to say on the subject.

BOURGEAULT • Actually I would simply like to tell the story of one of my former students. She was 27 at the time and the mother of a little girl of five. She had enrolled in a master's course under my direction. One day, she came into my office and said, "I have something important to tell you." She confided in me the news that she had cancer.

IKEDA • You must have been stunned.

BOURGEAULT • I listened attentively until she had finished. Several months earlier, discovering a lump in her breast, she had consulted a doctor. Tests showed that she had cancer and needed immediate surgery. She pleaded with the doctor to give her time to accomplish one or two things she wanted to do at all costs before going into the hospital.

IKEDA • So young . . . she must have been very shaken up. What was it she wanted to do before her surgery?

BOURGEAULT • She had already planned to visit her parents the next weekend to complete the detailed outline of her master's thesis on her father's computer. She delivered it to me the following Monday, adding as she did so, "Now I'm going into the hospital."

IKEDA • When her doctor informed her of her cancer, she made a reasoned judgment about how to proceed. I assume you are telling me that being informed had beneficial effects.

BOURGEAULT • Exactly. I had the feeling that she needed some time—a weekend with her parents—to carry out her projects. We could interpret this as a phase of denial before she became able to evaluate and cope with her new situation and the consequences of her cancer. The next time I had a chance to talk with her, she told me at length about what had happened in the meantime. She told me that her hospitalization had greatly saddened her daughter.

IKEDA • That was natural. Though only for a short time, the child had to part from her mother. Explaining the nature of her mother's sickness to her must have been difficult.

BOURGEAULT • That stands to reason. Some time later, the little girl asked, "Mummy, have you really told me everything?" Her mother said she had. Then, as she bathed her daughter, she explained how serious her condition was: "We all hope it won't happen, sweetheart, but Mummy might even die from this." Strangely enough, the girl was reassured by being candidly told the whole truth about her mother's condition.

IKEDA • A child of five may understand her mother's suffering, but at that age we can't really understand the meaning of death. Nonetheless, the girl was probably reassured: her mother was honest with her and treated her like a responsible individual. The fact that the child was reassured is testimony to the woman's profound love for her daughter and to the strong bond of mutual confidence between them.

BOURGEAULT • After her surgery, the young mother underwent all kinds of treatment for two or three years. She fought the disease with all the courage and energy she could muster, but eventually the cancer reappeared. All the while, she drew sketches to explain the progress of the illness to her daughter. As she was quite skilled at drawing, she produced a kind of illustrated narrative.

IKEDA • What a splendid way to communicate with a young child! Only a mother's love could have inspired such an ingenious method. She realized that it would be impossible to talk to her child about the disease and its symptoms using medical and biological jargon.

BOURGEAULT • The illustrated narrative was published a few months before its author died. In the story, a terrifying monster often appears in a child's bad dreams. The child weeps and cries out for her mother. Then suddenly, in the midst of a nightmare, a marvellous dragon appears and confronts the monster. He promises the child everlasting protection because, as he explains, "I am here in your heart."[11]

IKEDA • I am touched by the closeness of mother and child in their battle against a formidable illness. I am sure that the woman felt her vitality swelling and growing as she drew the illustrations for her daughter. In some sense, she probably also wanted to show her daughter how people can lead a courageous battle to overcome suffering. She used her own fight with cancer as an example.

11. Sophie LeBlanc in collaboration with Natacha LeBlanc-Filion. *Dragon in my heart.* Montreal: MNH Inc./Cedars Breast Clinic. 1997.

The *Path of the Law Sutra* (*Dhammapada*) says: "Heedfulness is the path to the Deathless . . . The heedful do not die." The mother and daughter battled together against the sufferings of sickness and death. Their battle became the "cause" in the life of the daughter that led to the "effect" of a lifelong ability to triumph over hardship.

BOURGEAULT • As a matter of fact, for several years before she became ill, the mother had been a Buddhist adherent. After her mother's speech at the launching of the book, the daughter took the microphone and said simply, "Thank you all for coming to this party for the publication of my mother's book." She was seven or eight at the time.

New kinds of suffering

IKEDA • This declaration of triumph on the part of mother and daughter has all the grandeur of an artistic masterpiece. It shows us that some children at that age are aware of the meaning of death. Surely this little girl, who confronted death with her mother, was more deeply aware than other children her age.

The death of their mother is perhaps the most mentally and emotionally stressful event for children to experience. How the child overcomes that stress—and in each case it is different—has a determining effect on the rest of the child's life. Some years ago Dr. Hans Selye (1907–82), former director of the Institute for Experimental Medicine at the University of Montreal, became widely known for his research on the topic. In fact, he was the first person to establish the concept of stress in the medical field.

BOURGEAULT • The work Dr. Selye and his team did on stress was certainly decisive. People sometimes consider stress a sickness of our times. In this connection I think it is useful to clarify two points. First—and the work of Dr. Selye was very revealing in this regard— strictly speaking, stress is not an illness or even a cause of illness. It mobilizes energies necessary for self-defense, self-protection, even creativity. Second, because all situations entail risk and present challenges, they are all stressful.

IKEDA • People are exposed on a daily basis to all sorts of situations— not only exterior circumstances like heat and cold, but psychological factors like anxiety and fear—that bring on systemic stress. Trouble in our personal and social lives can also be stressful. Indeed, in our time, psychological and social stress factors are becoming increasingly serious.

By assigning point values to stress factors in daily life, the American scientist Dr. T. Holmes (1918–88) came up with some highly interesting data. On a scale of 100, he set a value of 100 for the stress caused by the death of a spouse. Divorce was rated at 73 points, separation 65, and illness 53. Getting married, too, is stressful; Holmes gave it 50 points. Losing a job gets 47 points, being transferred 36, and new or changed work responsibilities 29. According to Holmes's study, 79% of the people with over 300 stress points within a year complained of some kind of physical or mental sickness.

BOURGEAULT · In psychogenic syndromes, influences reciprocate. That is to say, the body influences the spirit, and the psychological state affects physical condition.

IKEDA · The oneness of body and mind is one of the central tenets of Buddhism.

BOURGEAULT · A two-way movement is implied in the recognition of the psychosomatic nature of many complaints and illnesses. We often emphasize the influence of the mental state on the physiological state. We rely on psychological treatment—in the psychoanalytical tradition or some other school—to re-establish biological harmony or balance in a human being we recognize as a unit, rather than something compartmentalized according to various disciplines and specialties.

But the inverse is equally true. Physiological complaints—that is, dysfunctioning of the organism or sickness—can cause, or at least nourish and support, what the ancients called melancholy and what we today call depression. Violent or tenacious stress can provoke or aggravate stomach ulcers. Since this is the case, cannot stomach ulcers resulting from a faulty digestive system give rise to stress or cause it to increase? Human beings cannot escape stress. As long as we live, we must cope with it somehow. All life is full of stress.

IKEDA · The *Lotus Sutra* describes the threefold world (of desire, form and formlessness) as a burning house inhabited by unenlightened beings. It is said to be overflowing with the sufferings of mortal life—

birth, old age, sickness and death. In the Buddhist tradition, the fire represents anger, anxiety, fear, greed and other delusional desires.

BOURGEAULT · Today we can have no idea of the fears people once felt when lightning struck. They knew nothing of its origins or mechanisms, but it ripped off treetops and set forests ablaze. We do not know what they felt when famine threatened.

True, today new kinds of misfortune threaten and compromise human life, such as the complexity of the so-called developed societies you mentioned. Certainly this complexity is the source of many kinds of stress. To the usual list, I should like to add the current globalization of production and trade, economic globalization that causes pervasive unemployment. Fear of the future, which young people think is closed to them because they have no access to the job market and cannot find a place in the attractive social dynamic of adult life. People over 50 resent the lack of access to jobs because of business restructuring and forced early retirement. Felix Leclerc (1914–88) sings of one hundred thousand ways to kill a man. The easiest and most effective—perhaps the most brutal—is to refuse him the possibility—thus the right—to work, "to make a living." This is a pregnant expression because it describes the meaning of work and its connection with the quality of human life. Our societies make work a privileged, practically exclusive mechanism for social integration and yet shut out large groups, thus condemning them to marginalization or exclusion.

Precarious jobs. Poorly paid jobs. Unemployment. Are these not some of the causes of rising suicide rates—in Quebec, to stick to my own home ground—and of other kinds of violence in many countries undergoing "industrial restructuring" (to resort to a cynical euphemism)?

Stress is the spice of life

IKEDA · As you know, unstable social conditions, like those prevailing during economic downturns such as the ones experienced in Japan and throughout Asia over the past several years, have increased suicide rates among the middle-aged and elderly and violence among the young.

BOURGEAULT • When such things happen, there is a sudden proliferation of spiritual movements promising deliverance from all evils. Esoteric teachings inspired by these movements propose religious practices that claim to provide deliverance from evil. While I generally agree with your position on compassion and the importance of gratitude, I allow myself some reservations about certain psychological and religious trends that "disarm" combatants—if I may use the expression—and demobilize them, ultimately prompting passive toleration of everything, even the intolerable.

I just referred to the positive dynamic of stress as an instrument mobilizing energies to encourage self-defense. These same energies stimulate the creation of and commitment to concrete actions to redress, for instance, situations of injustice. In such instances, should spiritual practices free us of stress? And, if they succeed in this liberation, whose interests do they serve? Without being simplistic, I want to point out the ambiguity of practices that, under the pretext of helping people and improving their quality of life and their health, threaten to imprison them in unbearable situations and unacceptable conditions. To avoid misunderstanding, I should say that I recognize that some practices can help control stress and, above all, rechannel energy in creative, instead of destructive, directions.

IKEDA • I agree. We must have the wisdom to distinguish what is genuine from what is fraudulent. We must never allow ourselves to be taken in by fakes. Swallowing cleverly worded publicity and persuasive words can lead to unhappiness. Yet people still fall for such things and, rather than reinforcing their strength to deal with the challenges of modern life, grasp pitifully at the hope that one doubtful practice or another will vanquish their suffering. Suffering only gets worse when we try to run from it rather than facing it.

BOURGEAULT • You are right. One of Dr. Selye's most important contributions was to shed light on the positive aspects of stress. He argued that stress itself is not a sickness nor does it necessarily lead to sickness. It can enable us to exercise creativity and muster the vitality or energy we need to defend ourselves from exterior menace.

IKEDA • Dr. Seyle once described stress as "the spice of life." You really need to be free from worldly concerns to actually appreciate stress like that. It is healthy, and even necessary, to let go of the pressures of work and go have a drink with friends, sing in a karaoke bar or relax with some other form of recreation. Fundamentally, however, the important thing is to gather our internal forces enough to make stress a "spice" and to learn to use it creatively.

BOURGEAULT · The world of human beings is certainly no utopia of universal justice and peace. On the contrary, it is rife with injustice, discord and conflict. We must learn to live with these painful realities.

IKEDA · I held several discussions with the famous French biologist René Dubos, and he said that though it is pleasant to imagine a world free of worry, stress, and tension, such a world is no more than the pipedream of the indolent. He added that human beings develop in the face of adversity. This is how our spirits work—it is the destiny of humankind. What you just said reminds me of Dubos's words.

The most effective way to deal with stress is to constantly struggle to cultivate our minds and forge our personalities, even in the face of danger.

BOURGEAULT · No matter how absurd or irrational our circumstances, we can and must persevere in efforts to convert war into peace. Like liberty, equality and fraternity, justice and peace constantly elude us. We must nevertheless continue to make sustained efforts and to move, step by step, toward this unattainable goal and achieve at least fragments of peace and justice.

IKEDA · On the basis of his own experience fighting against cancer, Dr. Selye recommends the following in building a constructive life style: (1) Since resentment and anger lower one's resistance to stress, turn those feelings into respect and sympathy; (2) set goals for yourself; and (3) live for the benefit of others, for in so doing, you yourself will benefit.

The way of life Dr. Selye encourages is exactly what is called the bodhisattva way in Buddhism. Bodhisattvas live for the peace of humankind and to build a just and fair society. By so doing, they transform their indignation into compassion and control greed with wisdom. They enjoy their lives by making stress the spice of their vitality. A passage in the *Lotus Sutra* reads, "Jewelled trees abound in flowers and fruit where living beings enjoy themselves at ease."[12]

BOURGEAULT • Such qualities as vitality, self-control, creativity, wisdom, and perseverance are essential to the realization of justice and peace.

Again, it is not possible to totally avert war and completely eliminate injustice. But we can change the status quo; in fact, it is our duty to do so. At the very least, we are obligated to improve the realities of this world.

IKEDA • I agree absolutely.

BOURGEAULT • SGI has been working for years in close collaboration with the major agencies of the United Nations, including UNESCO. As president of SGI, you support the sentiment expressed in the opening of the UNESCO charter: "That since wars begin in the minds of men, it is in the minds of men that the defenses of peace must be constructed."

Building justice and peace day by day requires mobilization of energies of self-defense, creativity, and clear, warm-hearted inventiveness. Often the effect of the spiritual movements that proliferate today—regardless of whether or not this is the intention—is to demobilize and eliminate responsibility. No doubt, as I have said, injustices and wars are unavoidable. They exist—they scream at us from our television sets. But we can change things. It is our responsibility to do so or at least to work to that end.

IKEDA • True. The way to lasting peace is to make our minds firm citadels of peace even under the worst circumstances. I am convinced that this is the way to build the "human security" advocated by the United Nations.

6. Coping with Mental Illness

The importance of friends

IKEDA • Let us now turn to the problem of mental illness, the archetypal illness of the modern world, so closely related to the question of

12. *The Lotus Sutra*. Tr. Burton Watson. New York: Columbia University Press. 1993. 230.

stress. Specialists in Japan report increasing numbers of cases of depression. Indeed, it has become so frequent that some doctors call it the "mental common cold." Schizophrenia, too, is on the rise and has been described as a mirror of the contemporary social environment.

BOURGEAULT • In Canada, depression and schizophrenia are among the most common mental disorders. Until recently, various mental illnesses were indiscriminately lumped together under the categories of insanity and dementia. More precise diagnosis, however, has revealed the large variety of states observable today.

IKEDA • In other words, progress in medical science has made it possible to differentiate between conditions like schizophrenia and manic-depression.

BOURGEAULT • Exactly. But, although progress has undeniably been made in diagnosis, the same cannot always be said for treatment. In Canada, especially in Quebec, better knowledge of mental illness has convinced us to abandon the practice of keeping patients capable of fitting into society in specialized psychiatric institutions—once called insane asylums. But because of reductions in public funding allocated to health during the eighties and especially the nineties, essential community services are often lacking. Many itinerants and homeless, whose lot is certainly unenviable, suffer from mental-health problems and are left without support and often without medication.

IKEDA • How effective is medication for mental problems?

BOURGEAULT • Lithium carbonate has proven effective in controlling manic-depression, up to a point. But as far as I know, we still do not have really effective medicines against schizophrenia, although we can reduce some of its symptoms.

IKEDA • What therapies other than medication are being used against psychosis?

BOURGEAULT • Experiments with halfway houses, where a number of people suffering from mental-health problems live together under the supervision of a specialist, are being tried with reasonable success. The goal is progressive reintroduction into society. I am thinking specifically about experiments conducted in collaboration with various professionals (doctors, psychologists, and social workers—often women) at the Douglas Hospital in Montreal.

IKEDA • How effective were the halfway houses as therapy?

BOURGEAULT • I have known several people with experience in halfway houses. One came out fairly well, the others much less so. Still, their lives might have been even harder without the support they were afforded there.

Two of the people I personally knew succeeded in completing their university studies. One did so thanks to permanent medication and to his research advisor, who helped keep him on track. The other person rejected all medication and forced herself to remain in contact with "reality" by taking notes on her surroundings. Apparently, she wanted to preserve her dreamlike—or virtual—life. Though it was possibly more frightening than real life, it was also evidently more exciting. Of course, these people did not have easy lives. Among other things, they had difficulty establishing relationships that fit in with their own needs and expectations.

IKEDA • Auditory hallucinations and thinking disturbances often occur in schizophrenics. As I understand it, it is important for such people to have friends who treat them as equals. They need to be able to converse with people they can confide in spontaneously and honestly.

BOURGEAULT • Exactly. It is vital for friends and acquaintances to fully understand the condition of a mentally disturbed person. No matter what the treatment, responsibility for the consequences—or at least for some of them—must be shared with others. The support and understanding of friends, family—in fact, of everybody else—are crucial, although even they do not ensure success.

IKEDA • Understanding and responsibility are two qualities essential to any relationship based on trust. Certain Buddhist scriptures teach the fundamental ethics of personal relationships.

BOURGEAULT • What do they teach?

IKEDA • Well, as the old saying goes, "A friend in need is a friend indeed"—in other words, a good friend offers help in time of trouble. Such a friend is as true in hard times as in good times. True friends always have your best interests at heart in their dealings with you. And true friends always demonstrate care, compassion and sympathy. The sick have special need of such good friends.

The sutra also describes bad friends. These people take without giving—sometimes unwittingly. They are full of empty words and flattery, companions in dissipation. These people will never be true friends.

Relating to people

IKEDA • In the fall of 1997, I had the great good fortune to meet Dr. Linus Pauling, Jr. (1925–). He is a psychiatrist practicing in Hawaii. Dr. Pauling told me that, although cases of serious mental disorder are not increasing, growing numbers of people are becoming incapable of adapting to social, professional and family life.

BOURGEAULT • Our society does not facilitate the integration of people with mental-health problems. To function properly in society today—to work and to take part in social life—we must master abstract concepts and complex codes. Even people with outstanding qualities and diverse skills can be marginalized.

IKEDA • The wholesome development of society requires us to accept and make use of all kinds of human individualities, skills and qualities.

BOURGEAULT • That is very true. The people I was speaking of are full of talent! But the capacity for love, sadness, laughter and sympathy are hardly valued in today's pragmatic, highly competitive society.

IKEDA • Yes, I agree with you. Dr. Pauling and I discussed several aspects of human relations, including parent-child and teacher-pupil relationships. I shared with him the fourfold Buddhist concept of personal relationships, called *shi-shobo* in Japanese.

BOURGEAULT • What does that mean?

IKEDA • It refers to four ways of fostering the capacity to do good, to avoid evil and to follow the Middle Way. First is almsgiving, both material and spiritual, that relieves the other person's anxieties and imparts courage. Second is kind words, or using caring, compassionate speech. Third is benefiting others with good conduct in thought, word and deed, which means putting yourself in the other person's shoes. Fourth is an identification with others, the act of working and sharing with others. It seems to me that the ability to relate to others in these four ways is of growing importance in our increasingly technological and industrial society.

BOURGEAULT • I think so, too.

IKEDA • Dr. Pauling was very interested in this fourfold concept. He said that in the field of psychiatry, doctors have very particular relationships with their patients. The idea of almsgiving is applicable because of the supreme necessity for the doctor, in daily practice, to eliminate or reduce the patient's anxiety. The three other aspects of speech, benefit and shared identity could help patients discover other avenues of expression, new values and a new way of living and so achieve their full potential.

If "kind words" are used in discussions and conversations with patients, they will adopt more positive and constructive attitudes. Through dialogue, the psychiatrist also encourages patients to consider the emotions of others and make judgments from standpoints other than their own. Dr. Pauling explained that in the context of group therapy, it is impossible to avoid working closely and sharing with others. By grouping together patients with similar problems, doctors encourage them to share their opinions and feelings. In the process, many of them find the solutions to their personal problems.

BOURGEAULT • People stigmatized by mental-health problems are not the only ones who need the support of the groups they belong to. Or perhaps I should say that the difficulty the mentally ill experience is caused in part by the lack of such support and by the fact of being marginalized.

Personally, for more than twenty-five years I have relied on the support of a group that meets almost once a month to share a meal and exchange ideas. We impose only two rules. First, the host never provides the meal. Each person brings one dish. That way, everyone feels freer and more relaxed. Second, during the exchanges of ideas and discussion, we may be critical but we must never "judge," we must never make decisions for each other. We do not try to convince each other. Sometimes confrontations occur, but they are stimulating confrontations.

IKEDA • In the Soka Gakkai, we have long held similar discussion meetings. They are held in all countries, on the community or neighborhood level. Friends and acquaintances get together at someone's home to debate, discuss issues or study Buddhist teachings. Participants also give testimonials about the efficacy of faith. For many people, these meetings have a deeply therapeutic value. They are like a cure for heartache. But they don't feed the stomach—nobody brings food!

Human rights of the mentally disturbed

BOURGEAULT · In Canada, many people complain that mental illness and the mentally ill fail to receive the attention they deserve from governments, medical institutions, doctors, practitioners, and research workers. Very little is invested in mental illness—as if it were a shameful sickness. Is the situation the same in Japan?

IKEDA · In Japan, too, much less attention is paid to mental illness than physical illness.

BOURGEAULT · If the president of a large business has a heart attack, presumably from overwork, everybody admires him.

IKEDA · The Japanese react the same way. After all, we are supposedly "economic animals."

BOURGEAULT · If he suffers from depression, on the other hand, that same company president conceals it, out of humiliation.

IKEDA · I am sorry to admit that the Japanese tend to react the same way.

BOURGEAULT · Few agencies or organizations defend the rights of the mentally ill. Public funds allocated for research in this area are pitifully insufficient in comparison with the enormous sums invested in products or technologies that promise revolutionary therapies for cardiac illnesses.

IKEDA · I can't help thinking that the criteria for diagnosing mental illness seem vague and even arbitrary.

BOURGEAULT · They are. All the more so—in the field of education, for example—because of the chameleon effect that leads students to conform to the professor's expectations in order to demonstrate their brilliance—or stupidity.

IKEDA • That is a very important principle in educational psychology. We must not label people. The Buddhist concept of three thousand realms in a single life-moment (*ichinen-sanzen*), which I mentioned earlier, teaches that what is truly important is the manifestation of the individual's life at each moment, not what others think.

BOURGEAULT • Our self image is partly constructed from the opinions of others and above all by dominant social perceptions. Perceptions of health and the criteria by which it is defined vary from one society to another. What I call the "canons of normalcy," too, vary. We declare anyone who does not conform to those canons to be ill or handicapped.

IKEDA • Quite right. Our apparent criteria of normalcy and abnormality cannot be definitive.

BOURGEAULT • This is one of the major—and rarely discussed—issues of the development of biotechnologies, specifically genetic therapy. Research and experimentation in this field touches on what I—and others—call "soft eugenics." By this we mean eugenics that stops short of sterilizing people judged abnormal or, of course, exterminating them in gas chambers as the Nazi regime did in many countries during the thirties. Advocates of soft eugenics speak of redressing or restoring the so-called normal and "ordained" order. But who decides, and on what basis? In reference to what model of humanity?

IKEDA • The Buddhist concept of the mutual possession of the ten worlds (*jikkai-gogu*) teaches us that every life state or life condition is inherent in all others, from Hell right through to Buddhahood. In individual terms, a good person may at any moment become evil, and an evil person may demonstrate goodness.

BOURGEAULT • We are far from a sound understanding of the functioning of the brain and what is called the human spirit. Nonetheless, we can hope that progress in research will allow us to cure or comfort people afflicted with mental-health problems.

IKEDA • Your words will encourage many people. In addition to conducting research, we must eliminate social and economic discrimination against mental illness. We must build a society that recognizes and vigorously protects the rights of the mentally ill, the elderly, the handicapped, minorities, the socially underprivileged, women, and children. We must progress toward a human rights society.

BOURGEAULT · I doubt—and lament—however, that the rights of the mentally ill and society's treatment of them will become major issues in bioethics.

7. The Ideal Life

Reformers working for the sake of the people

IKEDA · Having discussed true good health from many angles, now, at the conclusion of this chapter on health and harmony, I should like to examine the optimum and healthiest way to live. In other words, I want to examine the ideal way of life. Dr. Bourgeault, who do you think has led an ideal life?

BOURGEAULT · To my way of thinking, no one has ever known an ideal life. We are all doomed to live the life given us, even when it sometimes contradicts our aspirations. We try to give meaning to it by taking strange detours.

Having said this, as a person interested in ethics and education, I immediately think of Socrates (470–399 BCE) and Jesus. And of Gandhi (1869–1948) and Martin Luther King Jr. (1929–68)—indeed, of everyone who has broken established rules and stood up against the authorities of their time, not capriciously but in the name of a strictly ethical imperative.

IKEDA · It's true. In keeping with the laws of his country, Socrates drank the poisoned cup when his sentence was pronounced. Jesus was crucified because of a confrontation with the authorities in his country. Both Mahatma Gandhi and Martin Luther King were assassinated in their non-violent combat against injustice.

BOURGEAULT · Each one of them knew exactly what awaited them if they publicly criticized the authorities or persisted in resisting the established powers.

IKEDA · You have singled out reformers, people willing to fight established authority and powers to save the ordinary people.

BOURGEAULT · It is now my turn to ask whom you respect most among the great figures of Buddhist tradition.

IKEDA · Mahatma Gandhi embodied the spirit of Buddhism better than anyone. This is why many of my Indian friends consider him the spiritual heir of Shakyamuni, who struggled against the corrupt ruling Brahman priests of his time twenty-five centuries ago. Gandhi advocated non-violent resistance (*ahimsa*) against Britain, the greatest empire of the day. As a Buddhist, I look at Gandhi in the same way.

In Japan, the person who best embodies the spirit of Buddhism was Nichiren Daishonin (1222–82), whose teachings I follow. Without the support of any secular authority, he addressed a letter of remonstration—*On Establishing the Correct Teaching for the Peace of the Land* (*Rissho Ankoku Ron*),[13]—to the Kamakura shogunate, which held absolute authority over the people at the time.

BOURGEAULT · What arguments did he advance?

IKEDA · He argued that, if the leaders of the nation ignored the fundamental law of the dignity of life (in conformance with the correct teaching), the people would suffer, hardships would arise, and society would collapse. The Daishonin urged the rulers to prevent this and to protect the country by making the well-being of the people the basic premise of government.

BOURGEAULT · I imagine his words were not well received!

IKEDA · Of course not. After he had delivered this remonstrance, the shogunate began to restrict his activities. He was arrested several times on false accusations, sentenced to death without trial, and exiled on an isolated northern island off the coast of Japan.

In spite of continuous and cruel persecutions, Nichiren continued the struggle, without giving an inch. Finally, in February 1274, the shogunate released him from exile. His predictions of catastrophe, civil war and invasion by foreign armies had all come true or were on the point of coming true. The first Mongol invasion occurred in October of the same year, in a massive military attack against the islands off Kyushu. At that point, the government had no choice but to heed Nichiren's warnings.

13. *The Writings of Nichiren Daishonin. 6.*

Upon returning to Kamakura, he said, "Even if it seems that, because I was born in the ruler's domain, I follow him in my actions, I will never follow him in my heart."[14] These words embody the Daishonin's determination never to be enslaved by the powerful. They might exile him, they might execute him, but they could not control his beliefs. He remained faithful to this conviction throughout his life.

Prizing life above all

BOURGEAULT · Such is the indomitable freedom of the prisoner. Recent history provides us with many similar examples. The environment, however, can support, threaten or weaken that freedom.

IKEDA · Incidently, those words of Nichiren Daishonin appear in a collection of famous quotations about human rights published to commemorate the twentieth anniversary of the founding of UNESCO.

The most powerful authority cannot enchain the heart and spirit. The voice of freedom cannot be stifled. I have relayed these words to intelligent and learned people all over the world, and today many are coming to see Nichiren Daishonin's life as an example of the struggle against authority for the sake of human rights. Tsunesaburo Makiguchi, the first president of Soka Gakkai, and my mentor Josei Toda, the second president, inherited the struggle and launched a movement that has not stopped growing.

BOURGEAULT · I have heard tell of their resistance to the Japanese government during World War II.

IKEDA · They were imprisoned by the military regime in 1943 on the pretext of having violated the Peace Preservation Law and for lèse-majesté because of their active opposition to the regime's policy of war. Makiguchi died in prison in November of the next year, at the age of 73. In a letter to his family, he wrote, "I'm doing quite well here in hell." He never stopped resisting authority. Inheriting Makiguchi's mission, Toda rose up alone, in the burned-out ruins of postwar Japan, to devote himself fully to the ordinary people.

14. *Ibid.* 579.

BOURGEAULT • People often say that life is what is most important. It seems self-evident. But Socrates, Gandhi, King, and many others considered it more important to preserve the meaning they assigned to their lives than to preserve their lives.

IKEDA • Very aptly put. Martyrdom is the fundamental spirit of religion. Nichiren Daishonin declared that "Life is the foremost of all treasures."[15] He taught that all the treasures of the universe together are worth less than life. He stressed his absolute belief in the sacred quality of life, and then added: "Fish want to survive; they deplore their pond's shallowness and dig holes to hide in, yet tricked by bait, they take the hook. Birds in a tree fear that they are too low and perch in the top branches, yet bewitched by bait, they too are caught in snares. Human beings are equally vulnerable. They give their lives for shallow, worldly matters but rarely for the noble cause of Buddhism."[16] In other words, preoccupied by self-interest, over-eager to protect their material circumstances, people lose their lives out of an obsession with greed and power. Nichiren didn't mince his words in denouncing the idiocy of human selfishness.

BOURGEAULT • The fish metaphor is very vivid.

IKEDA • The real question is to know, as you said, how we should live and what goals we should pursue if we want to honor the dignity of our lives. As Nichiren Daishonin expressed it, "Since nothing is more precious than life itself, one who dedicates one's life to Buddhist practice is certain to attain Buddhahood."[17] Alms or offering, in the Buddhist sense, means putting ourselves at the service of others. The Daishonin taught that struggling to protect the lives of others is the essence of nobility, both for ourselves and for others.

Helping people escape suffering, doing our best to support others, committing ourselves to improving communities and society at large, these are the most noble of human works. Along the way, we are bound to clash with those in power—those who lust after dominance. Lives may be lost in the fray. Such loss of life is martyrdom.

15. *Ibid.* 1125.
16. *Ibid.* 301.
17. *Ibid.* 301.

Despite this, I believe that the only way of life worthy of our humanity is to fight for the sake of world peace and the protection of human rights. A life dedicated to these noble goals radiates a light of its own. This is the bodhisattva way embodied by the bodhisattva Vimalakirti I spoke of earlier. His acceptance of responsibility for others' pain makes him a perfect example of humanity in its full splendor.

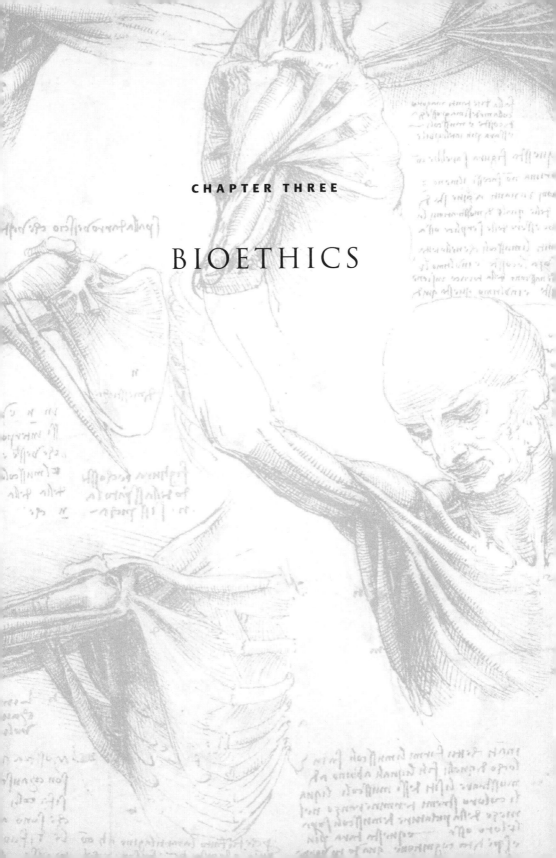

CHAPTER THREE

BIOETHICS

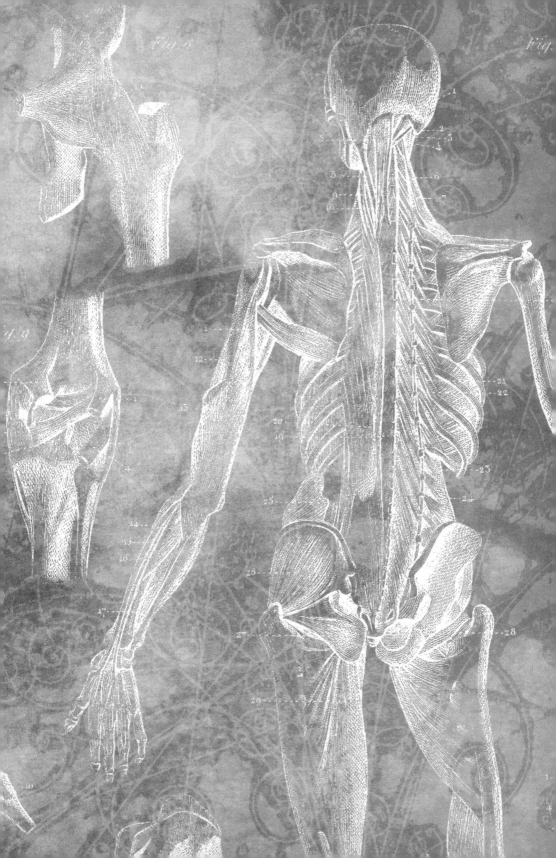

1. Religion and Medical Ethics

The values that inspire Western medicine

IKEDA • Buddhism arose from humankind's struggle to overcome the most fundamental problems of human existence—the four sufferings of birth, aging, sickness, and death. These four conditions—though sources of pain—are inseparable from human life. The confrontation with these problems is also expressed as Shakyamuni's "four encounters." Witnessing the effect on humans of old age, sickness, death and religious faith, Shakyamuni abandoned secular life to seek a way to overcome the four sufferings.

Shakyamuni's efforts both to come to terms with these conditions that continue throughout the chains of human existence and to attain happiness are still a fundamental task for humanity. Even after Shakyamuni's death, the teachings of Buddhism are still centered on its concern with the four sufferings.

The immense philosophical canon known as the *Abhidharma* (doctrinal studies and commentaries on the sutras) includes a book called *A Treasure of Analyses of the Law* that examines the four sufferings from many angles, based largely on contemporary medical knowledge—notably the wisdom of the *Sacrificial Prayer Veda*. What are your thoughts, Dr. Bourgeault, on the relationship between birth, death, and sickness on the one hand and religion on the other?

BOURGEAULT • I must first make it clear that I am not a religious man. Although I have studied the Bible and Christian theology, I am certainly not a representative of any Christian church and not even a believer. Still, the Judeo-Greco-Christian origins of ideas about life and death, health and sickness are obviously generally—if vaguely—accepted in North America and Europe.

Health policies, for example, go back, sometimes explicitly, more often implicitly, to the grand ideas of liberty, equality, and fraternity that were the rallying points of the American Revolution of 1775–83 and the French Revolution of 1789, the declarations of which still inspire democracies in North America and Europe. These secular ideas recognize the dignity of every human being as a right. They dispute both political and religious despotic powers, establishing a social contract that creates among all members of a given society a solidarity expressed in mutual respect for others and responsibility for the weakest members. And they strive to harmonize the rights of the group with the rights of each individual.

These ideals are clearly rooted in the Christian tradition, especially in the teachings of Jesus and Paul, who were themselves heirs of older traditions. Jesus contested established laws and hierarchies and called for solidarity and compassion for the poor in a utopian society where the liberty of the children of God would create egalitarian relationships of mutual understanding and assistance. In his own way, Paul continued this vision by contesting artificial distinctions and divisions between men and women, free people and slaves, Jews and non-Jews.

Contemporary health and health services policies come under the banner of individual dignity and the right to freedom, by offering services to satisfy the individual right to health. They come under the sign of equality, by making these services accessible to every individual. Finally, they come under the sign of solidarity—if not fraternity—by making everybody, including the healthy, pay for services dispensed to the sick.

IKEDA • In other words, medical ethics is closely related to the concept of human dignity.

BOURGEAULT • In Europe and North America, the ethics of health professionals has long been characterized, on the one hand, by fundamental exigencies imposed by the dignity of individuals and the dignity of life—or their right to self-determination, as we would eventually come to say—and, on the other hand, by what is commonly called the principle of charity, which calls for preferential attention to be accorded the poor and the sick. This attention is often cited as a characteristic of Christian solidarity.

According to the Gospels, Jesus was resolutely on the side of the poor, the sick, the marginalized, and the socially excluded. He took up their cause and made service to neighbors, the poor, and the sick a sign of belonging to a new humanity. The "good news"—or gospel—was the announcement that the poor, the ill, the sick, and the outcasts would occupy primary places in the Christian community. Stories of miraculous cures illustrate this. Medical care and professional support for the sick are included in the compassionate, restorative and miraculous actions of Jesus.

IKEDA • The Judeo-Christian spirit was of course influenced by contacts with the classical spirit.

BOURGEAULT • Yes. We cannot understand the origins and development of professional medical ethics in Europe, and later in the United States, without taking into account their Greco-Roman roots. Today medical ethics codes are still founded on the Hippocratic Oath, which dates to the fourth century BCE.

The encounter between the Judeo-Christian and Greco-Roman heritages leads us to think of human action as co-creationist and oriented toward remaking the world by filling in the gaps of creation, correcting its "errors," "curing" people and freeing them from their pain. As I have already said, it is scarcely surprising that Western medicine progressively concentrates more on the battle to conquer illnesses like cancer and AIDS than on greeting and accepting illness in what Buddhism calls—if I understand correctly—inner harmony or wisdom.

Harmony of body and mind, life and environment:
The Buddhist view of health

IKEDA • We could say that Christianity adopts the view of sickness as an external enemy that must be overcome. As you point out, Buddhism, on the other hand, sees illness as a matter of discord between the body and the spirit and between life and its environment. The Buddhist approach promotes health by reinforcing the "dynamic harmony" inherent in life. It ceaselessly pursues what is now called quality of life, a central consideration in modern bioethics.

BOURGEAULT · What kind of quality of life does Buddhism teach?

IKEDA · Buddhism proposes three main ways of improving the quality of life. The first is precepts (*kai*). Precepts concern the ability to take control of insatiable desires and channel them in the right direction. This is the foundation of autonomy.

Second is the constant search for universal truth (*jo*). This means permanency or regularity in a world where people are continuously contraried and beset with vicissitudes. Constancy, or permanence, describes the unshakeable determination to find and uphold the truth, to always act in accordance with the truth, no matter what obstacles arise.

Third is practical wisdom founded on that universal truth (*e*). This idea expresses the unlimited potential for self-actualization present in all of us. When we acknowledge unlimited potential, we must be wise enough to recognize it in others as well as in ourselves. Enlightened recognition of infinite potential must be mutual, and must be acted upon. Buddhism urges us to integrate these three concepts— autonomy, permanence and practical wisdom—into our way of life, and in so doing, to raise our quality of life.

BOURGEAULT · To these key Buddhist concepts of autonomy, permanence and practical wisdom I should like to add dignity, individual rights, solidarity, fraternal support (or "brotherly love," to use traditional Christian terminology) and action to transform, repair, and even re-create the world.

IKEDA · Buddhist discipline, too, assumes the practice of autonomy, permanence and practical wisdom assumes the form of compassion, in connection with relationships with others. In this case, compassion means action taken to overcome the sufferings of life, together with other people, based on respect for their human dignity.

What kind of humanity do we want for tomorrow?

BOURGEAULT • In recent decades, scientific and technological developments have achieved stunningly audacious transformations in all fields of human endeavor, perhaps most strikingly in the field of biomedicine. This is why bioethics had to break new ground to replace outdated professional morals. Professional practices changed much earlier than the ethical framework. This happened principally because of a growing recourse to increasingly complex and precise technologies that paved the way for increasingly daring actions.

IKEDA • Medical ethics reform was unable to keep pace with revolutionary medical developments.

BOURGEAULT • New fields of treatment opened up—and new areas of questioning. This is exactly the function of bioethics, to intervene at a moment of rupture with the past. As has been observed, the lack or inadequacy of old morals and their inability to take the biomedical achievements of recent decades into consideration led us to break with them for the sake of exploring new paths.

IKEDA • That is why it is urgently necessary to create a new ethics compatible with the medical revolution and capable of guiding medical science.

BOURGEAULT • Bioethics represents an awareness—a will—to tackle new problems connected with the development and use of technologies in the biomedical field. It is not just an effort to update a code reserved exclusively for doctors or health professionals.

Bioethics proposes to address new and complex problems in a resolutely multidisciplinary fashion. It suggests dealing with them case by case through discussions in pluralist societies that do not ascribe to a pre-determined vision of the human being—discussions which can serve as a sure benchmark for deciding what should and should not be done.

IKEDA • Contemporary societies with increasingly diverse values all share the same kinds of problems.

BOURGEAULT • The human being is no longer perceived as a given but as something to shape. And we are constantly reshaping the human being at a steadily accelerating rhythm of ever-bolder actions. This is why we must debate the question that I raised earlier, the question that concerns everybody: now that the consensus of yesterday no longer holds, what kind of humanity do we want for tomorrow?

IKEDA • The nature of the humanity we want for tomorrow is the cardinal point of the new bioethics. We will need dialogue to create a new image of humankind.

BOURGEAULT • It is the duty and essential, democratic task of bioethics to stimulate public discussion of these fundamental issues, because ultimately they concern the lives of every one of us.

Partnership between patients and caregivers

IKEDA • Human relations at medical-treatment centers are an important bioethics issue. A particularly significant change has come about in the relationship between medical staff and patients, with a move from a tradition model of imposed authority to a more balanced model of shared responsibility. This new kind of relationship aims to make the patient an equal partner with the doctor. The importance of the right to self-determination and informed consent is now recognized. Dr. Bourgeault, what are your thoughts on this relationship from a medical-ethics point of view?

BOURGEAULT • Relations between doctors and other health professionals and the people who call on their services have evolved over the years. In a work on bioethics published some time ago,[1] I pointed out the great landmarks and dates that trace this evolution from the Hippocratic Oath—which I later compared to ancient Indian and Chinese texts—to such great contemporary declarations as those of the International Medical Association made at Helsinki (1964) and later at Tokyo (1975) and the more recent one of the World Health Organization.

From these texts it is easy to draw up relationship models that define doctors as "fathers," as experts, or as partners in a course of action they do not entirely and exclusively control.

Let me explain further.

1. *L'éthique et le droit face aux nouvelles technologies biomédicales* (Ethics, human rights and new biomedical technology). Brussels and Montreal: De Boeck-Wesmael/ PUM. 1990.

THE PATERNALIST MODEL. In societies where culture and all life depend on superior forces that dictate how things evolve, at times of crises people give precedence to the intervention of priests or sorcerers believed to be in contact with those superior forces. In the collective mind, doctors were long perceived to be the heirs to the secret, mysterious powers of priests and sorcerers. This paternalistic relationship prolonged the sacerdotal model in a secularized form. In this type of relationship, one party knows and the other doesn't, which leads the second party—the patient, in this instance—to recognize and submit to the undisputed and indisputable authority of the first—the doctor.

THE ENGINEER OR EXPERT MODEL. With the development of science and technology, all professionals—including health professionals—became in a sense "engineers." In recent years, denunciations have been made of medical practitioners who revert to a mechanistic, reductionist anthropology. Instead of regarding their patients as the primary agents in actions supported by others on the basis of their individual competencies, the doctor-engineer treats the patient as an object of isolated interventions, commanded from without.

IKEDA • The first two models are hierarchical relationships, whereas the third suggests equality.

BOURGEAULT • Yes, I call it THE PARTNERSHIP MODEL. The first two models I described are like photographic negatives of another model sometimes called a contractual relationship, though I prefer to call it a partnership. This model is part contract and part friendliness. The contract sets down the equality of the two parties; the friendliness expresses their close association in a fundamentally collaborative act— a human commonality, the responsibilities of which will be jointly accepted. This approaches the compassion of which you spoke, but without the religious dimension explicit in Buddhist tradition.

This model places the professional and the professional's actions in the dynamic of a conscious, deliberate partnership that orchestrates diverse, complementary efforts. Each party remains the primary agent of his or her own life. Each party determines his or her own orientation and makes the necessary choices. Each party takes appropriate action. Most important, each party defines "well-being" and "quality of life" on his or her own. Although this is done with the help of others, notably specialists or professionals, the patient maintains control of the whole process from beginning to end—from examination and situation analysis to reparative or curative action by way of diagnosis and therapy selection.

IKEDA • I also believe that the doctor and patient should face their tasks as partners, united in the effort to defeat disease. The idea reminds me of the Three Admonitions of Buddhist medicine—one to doctors, one to nurses, and one to patients—exhorting them to cooperate and learn together to battle against illness. In this way all can find fulfilment. Ethical demands are made of all three.

Nagarjuna's *Treatise on the Sutra of the Perfection of Wisdom* says the ideal doctor or "Grand Healer" should be skilled in the healing arts, full of compassion, and indifferent to the patient's financial condition. *The Great Canon of Monastic Rules* admonishes nurses to care for patients gently and compassionately, without thinking of personal advantage. It warns that thinking of personal gain destroys compassion. It also encourages patients to endure pain, live regular, disciplined lives, and acquire enough knowledge to understand their own conditions.

In general, these Buddhist medical ethics suggest approaching treatment and patient care as a shared and reciprocal effort to which doctor, nurse and patient all contribute.

2. Definition of Death

From God's will to human life and death

IKEDA • The first organ transplant in Japan took place in 1968, but it wasn't until 31 years later, in March 1999, two years after the enactment of the Organ Transplant Law, that another surgery involving vital organs took place. The first Japanese transplant operation—performed three decades earlier—was questionable from various viewpoints and was followed by a hiatus in organ donation surgeries in Japan.

The recent revival of transplants, however, has aroused great interest in brain death and death with dignity. To get to the basic premise of bioethics, I would like to discuss the nature of human life and the various ways people define death.

BOURGEAULT • For the past twenty years, pragmatic, decision-oriented bioethics as practiced in the United States and Canada has managed to achieve common consensus by avoiding all meaningful discussion of the most basic question: what is human life? I think it is about time to tackle this issue squarely and to simultaneously ask another question: what is human death?

IKEDA • That is a good point. In a lecture I gave in 1993 at Harvard University, I expressed my conviction that modern civilization has failed in its attempt to overlook death. To avoid looking at death is to neglect inquiries into the meaning of life. As you said, we try not to tackle the most important issue: life and death.

If we try to ignore death, death will insinuate itself anyway. We have only to look at the numerous instances of war and genocide in the twentieth century to see it. When we ignore the meaning of life, we end up undervaluing life. We see rampant violence today, and each act of violence shows how lightly we take life today.

BOURGEAULT • My own interest in ethical order has made me particularly mindful of widespread and constant violence against life and our astonishingly widespread irresponsibility toward it.

IKEDA • In a lecture you delivered in Japan, entitled "Science and Technology and the Responsibility of Humankind," you said that modern technoscientific progress has engendered an age in which both the global environment and human life itself are being disrupted by new kinds of change. As you point out, in the past the boundary between life and death was taken for granted. Modern ways of manipulating life, however, blur that boundary.

BOURGEAULT • Definitely. Even before birth, prenatal tests—pre-implantation tests in the case of in vitro fertilization—can determine the "quality" of life in store for the gestating embryo if it is allowed to develop. The emergence of new choices poses new questions. And this situation continues until the end of life. In the last moments, we can separate life from agonizing sufferings. We can hasten or delay death itself, whose ancient power, if not yet abolished, can be held temporarily in check. One cannot, however, avoid raising the question of the meaning of life, which becomes especially acute just before death.

IKEDA • Indeed, progress in modern medicine has reintroduced questions about the nature of life and death.

BOURGEAULT • I was born and raised in a society steeped in Christian tradition. All cultural traditions—often religious in nature—abound with ideas, images, myths, and metaphors that provide guideposts for our conduct in life. I am happy that we have been given a chance to set two great traditions—the Buddhist and the Christian—in parallel and perhaps in communion. I should like to take this chance to say that I read your article on brain death with great interest. I learned much about the Buddhist conception of death from it.

IKEDA • We will get to the subject of brain death later on. Right now I would like to ask you about the Christian idea of death. I believe Christianity teaches that death is the result of the will of God.

BOURGEAULT • Back when no one could change the course of life, or more specifically, the course of sickness, a priest would come quickly to take over from the doctor. A Christian prayer recited at the approach of death goes something like this, "The Lord giveth, and the Lord taketh away. Praise be to God." In other words, life is a gift from God; it is not mine. Therefore I am not free to end it or prolong it as I see fit.

IKEDA • But today medical science is deeply involved in prolonging human life and postponing death. Artificial respirators and intensive care units are used to prolong at death's door lives that, in the past, would already have ended. Since modern medicine is able to prolong life in these ways, we cannot deny its merits. But we must try to use its powers wisely. And this brings us back to the issue of the nature of death.

Three functional levels of life and the principle of nine consciousnesses

BOURGEAULT • It seems to me that in recent years we have been more concerned with defining the moment of death pragmatically than with discussing its meaning. The goal is to set guidelines, to help us decide whether to discontinue treatment and whether to proceed to harvesting and transplanting organs.

People are generally unaware of what has brought us to this juncture. I might refer back to ancient Greek anthropology, which distinguished between the body and the feelings, the psyche and the sentiments, the soul or the spirit and reason. In the Middle Ages, people fiercely debated the moment at which the human embryo is animated. They drew distinctions between the vegetable and animal kingdoms—both separate from human beings. In direct line with this tradition, people have recently distinguished various functional levels in human beings. First, biological functions like circulation and respiration, which keep the organism alive. Second, sensual functions and motion, which permit the living being to react to exterior stimuli. Third, functions of conscience and communication, which are specific to human beings. As the ravages of a sickness grow worse, it becomes doubtful whether human life persists when awareness seems extinguished, although the vital—that is, biological—functions continue.

If I am not mistaken, the Buddhist tradition posits a scale of levels of life comparable to the one I have just outlined.

IKEDA • To answer that, I would like to cite the Buddhist teaching that I think is most relevant to this three-stage concept. It is called the principle of the nine consciousnesses and it presents the Buddhist vision of the essence of life.

The first five levels of consciousness correspond to the five senses: sight, hearing, smell, taste, and touch. They are simply consciousness of the exterior world. The sixth level, known as the thinking spirit or "mental consciousness," integrates these five and passes judgment on the exterior world. This could be compared to what is called consciousness in Western psychological terminology.

The seventh level represents the internal, spiritual world (*mana* consciousness). This is the source of identity of the self, operating in the name of self-preservation and expansion. It seems to correspond to the Western idea of the ego.

The eighth level is called the *alaya* consciousness or "storehouse." On a deeper level, this eighth consciousness stores the energy that supports all the other consciousnesses. This energy is manifest in thought, word, deeds and emotion. This is where "karma" comes from. Jung's "collective subconscious" is the Western psychological counterpart of the *alaya* consciousness.

Some schools of Buddhism posit the existence of a ninth consciousness which is the true entity of life and the basis of all the other functions. Your three functional levels seem to correspond to the first seven Buddhist consciousnesses.

BOURGEAULT · Could you explain more specifically how they correspond?

IKEDA · In your first stage, there is neither sensitivity nor awareness. In Buddhist terms, this means that life activities are confined to the seventh consciousness or below. In your second level, the person reacts to pain and other stimuli, but is unable to communicate. Here the self-preservation aspects of the seventh consciousness are active, allowing the first five and sixth consciousnesses to perform according to their natures, but the activity is passive. In your third level, the person is able to interact with the exterior world in a positive and independent fashion. At this level, the five sensory consciousnesses and the sixth consciousness are fully functional.

BOURGEAULT · In the West, people tend to think that the capacities to know, judge, and communicate distinguish the human state from all others.

IKEDA · In other words, beings living in your third level are recognized as human while, if I understand you correctly, those living in levels one and two are something less.

BOURGEAULT · The distinctions are more nuanced and the problems more complex. Loss of conscience does not entail loss of the right to life. Since uncertainty persists about the moment at which death occurs, people have tried to establish guidelines to control removal of organs for transplantation. This led us to resort to the notion of brain death.

A continuing process

IKEDA • Earlier in my explanation of the nine consciousnesses, I made no distinction between human and non-human life. This is because Buddhism interprets life as a continuum. According to this line of thinking, at death, life moves progressively from the third level of full consciousness to the second level of residual sensitivity to external stimuli, and then on to the first level or comatose state in which no response is made to the external world. Moving from level three to level two is not considered a loss of humanity. Perhaps it is in this that the Buddhist view differs most noticeably from Western ideas.

BOURGEAULT • The West, too—especially in the face of the great ecological challenges of our times—is becoming aware of a continuity of life that motivates us to protect life in all its forms.

IKEDA • That view coincides with the Buddhist way of thinking. A person who manifests the seventh consciousness (deep subconscious) is still considered living, even though outside observers may be unaware of it. Such a person can still receive external information and stimuli and experience emotional reactions.

Nurses have told me some touching tales on the subject. One told me she had spoken softly to a comatose patient and played his favorite music. Upon regaining consciousness, he expressed his gratitude for her kind words and attentions. She was thrilled, of course, but also frankly astonished that he not only knew what was happening around him while he was in the coma, but that he was able to remember afterward.

The members of a medical team who treat presumably dying comatose patients mechanically or coldly would no doubt be mortified to hear recriminations from those patients should they regain consciousness. I would hate to be in their shoes!

Buddhist teachings assume continuity rather than segmentation of the stages of life.

BOURGEAULT • Perceiving life stages as a continuum might give us a new perspective on points of convergence between traditional Eastern and Western thought.

IKEDA • You are suggesting an interpretation of life deeper and more inclusive than traditional ones. In the Buddhist view, death is regarded as a passage through the three levels you described. It culminates in union between the eighth or *alaya* consciousness and the life of the cosmos itself. Brain death is one point in this process.

3. Brain Death

Responsibility and solidarity

BOURGEAULT • For a long time, human beings—as individuals and as a collective—have perceived themselves to belong to a universe far larger than themselves. They depend on its order and are subject to the natural laws and rules governing it. Scientific and technological developments of the last decades have been oriented toward the transformation of the world and its natural order and toward the modification of human life itself. They have introduced us to a new cultural universe. After a frenzy of grand projects to deconstruct and reconstruct the world—to transform life—growing unrest now calls urgently for a sense of responsibility.

IKEDA • Are you referring to each person's responsibility for his or her own life?

Shakyamuni explained the fundamental spirit of Buddhism as a sense of individual responsibility. "You are your only master. Who else? Subdue yourself and discover your master."[2] In other words, we must each take responsibility for our own self-discipline and for cultivating meaningful lives.

He goes on to say that we must each save ourselves. No child, no parent, no family member can face death for us. This means that, in clinical instances, each of us has the free will to determine whether to terminate or prolong our lives, to live as we judge best. Of course, agreement among family members and the cooperation of friends and doctors are essential. Nonetheless, the individual makes the final decision. This has been the Buddhist philosophy since the time of Shakyamuni.

2. The Path of the Law Sutra (*Dhammapada*), Volume XII.

BOURGEAULT • We envision the ethical issues at stake differently depending on whether we regard human life as a gift, a project, or an individual and collective responsibility. If life is a gift—moreover a divine gift—we regard it as intangible and afford it absolute respect from the beginning of embryonic existence to the last breath. We attempt neither to create it artificially nor to shorten its course when it seems to become meaningless. The meaning of life as a gift, with its unforeseen potentialities, is itself given. If we regard life as a personal project, on the other hand, it ceases to be apparent that we must not terminate it when the meaning we seek to impart to it proves unattainable. Finally, if we see life as part responsibility and part solidarity, we must take the social and political dimensions of our decisions into consideration, above and beyond our individual desires.

IKEDA • Technoscientific developments have made your first approach—leaving life and death entirely up to the will of God—no longer practical. The second approach—the personal project—consists largely of following the caprices of earthly desires. This may give an illusion of freedom, but it can degenerate into selfishness and self-indulgence and can bring on the ruin of the self and of others as well. That only leaves the third, the individual responsibility approach, the only way that honors the dignity of life.

BOURGEAULT • But the transition from a morality of duties or rights and liberties to an ethic of interdependent responsibility will not occur by itself.

IKEDA • Responsibility and solidarity are indeed the ethical model human beings must strive for. A passage in the Buddhist scriptures says, "Those who protect themselves protect others as well. Protect yourself and you will be wise and come to no harm" (*Anguttara Nikaya*). In other words, self-responsibility requires a sense of solidarity.

Buddhism further teaches that the self and the other are so closely related as to be inseparable. All beings exist solely in their relationship to each other. They are bound together by the law of dependent origination. They must therefore cooperate and seek happiness together. Seeking happiness only for one's self is doomed to failure. The only reasonable alternative is to join forces with each other for the good of all. This means that the person with a sense of self-responsibility also feels responsible for the lives of others and considers solidarity a duty.

BOURGEAULT • I think that an ethics of responsibility requires us not to reject innovation but to circumscribe its risks and to restrain its harmful effects as much as possible.

IKEDA • A most appropriate definition. The idea of brain death may require a new approach to mortality. Nonetheless, maximum consideration must be taken of any possible negative consequences. Everyone engaged in the debate has a responsibility to minutely examine all possible ramifications.

More precise criteria for the declaration of brain death

BOURGEAULT • According to medical practices authorized in Canada, the United States, and Europe, irreversible coma is considered a sign of brain death—thus the end of human life—and suffices for permission not only to terminate treatment, but also to remove organs for transplantation.

IKEDA • That seems to coincide with the current medical point of view.

BOURGEAULT • But can we legitimately and logically associate—or equate—an indication of death with a reality that escapes our perception and control? Can we in this way determine the moment when a human life—a life with human qualities—ceases, even though it continues to perform so-called vital functions? The problem, if I can put it this way, is that people no longer die naturally in hospitals. Instead, may die because they are "unplugged." Hospitals cannot serve as storehouses for people under deferred death sentence!

At what moment can we unplug a patient, or stop providing treatment deemed no longer useful? Who should make this decision? When, exactly, is a person dead and when should he or she be declared dead? Based on what criteria and what indications? And with what degree of certainty? What percentage of error is tolerable? Because there will no doubt be errors—which of course we won't even be aware of!

IKEDA · That is exactly the aspect of brain death that worries many people.

BOURGEAULT · We must propose an acceptable general framework and establish rules. Though it may seem cynical, we are compelled to talk in terms of risks and tolerable errors. We must realize that risks exist and determine under what conditions they are morally acceptable. In this connection, I will limit myself to the notion of moral certitude commonly in use first by European and then by American philosophers since the sixteenth century. Moral certitude is defined as the degree of certitude required and sufficient to ensure that the decision taken and its subsequent actions are themselves moral. This appears tautological, but the basic idea behind it seems just and important. We must know that the required and sufficient certitude has been reached after a faithful effort to understand and take into consideration all known elements in the problem or situation, even though we realize that we cannot know and master them all. In other words, we must recognize the possibility of a persisting incertitude.

The question of defining death and determining the moment of its occurrence is all the more pressing because every day people are making the decision to terminate the battle against death or to remove organs from what is considered a cadaver. Unable to give a totally certain answer to the first question—which refers back to the vexatious issue of defining life—we have nevertheless established parameters useful in medical practice in relation to the second question.

IKEDA · As we said earlier, the party involved must take the initiative beforehand for accepting medical judgment on brain death and state willingness to donate organs. In Japan, people often carry donor cards indicating agreement to these conditions. The nature of family participation in the decision is still being debated.

I agree that "moral certitude" is of the essence in this issue. A similar certitude is necessary for the patient and his or her family to accept the medical verdict of brain death and consent to organ donation. This is one way to minimize the negative effects of the decision.

BOURGEAULT · In Canada, the medically and legally recognized definition of brain death presupposes the total arrest of all cerebral functions, including those of the brain stem, which controls things like spontaneous respiration. Once brain death has been confirmed, it is permissible, with the consent of the relatives, to terminate treatment and proceed to remove organs.

Basing their approach on the thought of American and European philosophers, some people suggest we consider dead anyone whose superior cerebral functions—which enable consciousness and communication—have ceased. This would make greater supplies of organs available for transplantation. So far, their request has been unfavorably received.

IKEDA • Although the criteria may differ slightly, in Japan, too, we consider the cessation of all brain functions, including the brain stem, as the basis for determining brain death.

BOURGEAULT • Some people contest the validity of defining human death on the basis of brain death, denouncing a legal flaw in its objective. They argue that the purpose of the definition is to terminate treatment and more specifically to obtain organs for transplanting and that the definition of brain death has been "invented" or adjusted to authorize those practices. Personally, I cannot accept this. Although I recognize the ambiguity of the definition and the element of uncertainty it entails, I nonetheless consider the definition legitimate and useful for reasons already advanced: the need to act and the absence of certainty in spite of that need.

IKEDA • My article on brain death calls for more precise criteria and argues that society will accept brain death as a basis for judgment if it is proven that the functions of the entire brain are irretrievably lost, that is, if the damage is irreparable.

If we refer back to the three levels of life, this would mean people on the first level who have reached a point where medical science as we know it can no longer improve their condition. In terms of the nine consciousnesses, it means a state in which the five senses and the coordinating function provided by the sixth and seventh consciousnesses have been irretrievably lost.

That said, however, I hope that repeated debate from many vantage points will enable us to formulate a convincing moral certitude. We must found our decisions on ethical models that entail individual responsibility and a sense of solidarity with our fellow humans. The same mature consideration is needed to deal with the issue of transplanting organs from the brain dead.

By the way, are organ transplants frequent in Canada today?

BOURGEAULT • Organ transplants are fairly widespread in Canada. According to statistics compiled in 1991, more than 800 kidney transplants, 5 kidney-pancreas transplants, 144 heart transplants, 58 lung transplants, 10 heart-lung transplants, and 174 liver transplants were performed. For a transplant to take place, the donor must have clearly stated willingness. This may be done in written form—on a card that citizens are encouraged to carry with them for the sake of rapid action in case of accident—or it may be verbal, in which case, relatives, too, must give their consent.

IKEDA • With more than twenty years of history behind it, organ transplantation in Europe and North America is technically advanced. Rejection of the transplanted organ was once a great obstacle, but new drugs have solved this problem. Today many transplant recipients recover their health and lead normal lives.

In Japan, by contrast, no organ transplants were carried out for almost a year and a half after the law permitting them went into effect. This is partly because social consensus on brain death has yet to be achieved and partly because of a traditional Japanese belief that the body, living or dead, is the permanent seat of the soul. There have even been cases in which family objections have resulted in cancellations of planned transplants in spite of prior donor consent.

BOURGEAULT • In general, religious authorities approve transplants in the belief that they respect the dignity of the individual and—from the standpoint of the donor—are in line with the Christian dynamic of fraternity or solidarity—what you would no doubt call compassion. I would add that relatives often feel comforted in their mourning by the idea that the death of a beloved person has benefited someone else and that life thus triumphs over death.

IKEDA • We must all consider brain death and organ transplantation as personal issues. Families should discuss honoring each other's wishes in this connection.

Even in the West, where organ transplants are now routine, it took years to achieve social consensus. In Japan, we have a long way to go before discussions of the issue reach this level.

BOURGEAULT • An international network of information makes delivery of extracted organs possible—across national boundaries—to appropriate recipients. The system is not, however, without risk of such abuses as commerce in organs at the expense of the poor—individuals and whole peoples. There is no reason to think, however, that such abuses have been or are current in Canada, where standing laws clearly forbid commerce in human organs or tissues and all infringements of bodily integrity.

Still, organ removal and transplantation are complex, requiring the orchestrated cooperation of many performers. Of necessity, they are institutionalized and therefore subject to the play of exchanges, confrontations, and controls.

4. Death with Dignity: Overcoming the Suffering of Death

Buddhism condemns active and voluntary euthanasia

IKEDA • What are your thoughts on euthanasia and death with dignity?

BOURGEAULT • The news media frequently reopen the debate on euthanasia. As people say, "They shoot horses, don't they?" If that is so, why should we condemn human beings to suffer prolonged agony?

IKEDA • The meaning of the word *euthanasia* differs from one historic period and one nation to another. Here I refer to its most commonly accepted meaning: that is, the shortening of an incurably ill patient's life, on the basis of that patient's own will and the wishes of his or her family. I'm speaking of what can be called "compassionate murder," a deliberate intervention, in keeping with the wishes of the person involved, to hasten death in order to eliminate intolerable suffering.

BOURGEAULT • We sometimes still make a distinction between direct and indirect, or active and passive euthanasia. But the development of a techno-medical arsenal has rendered null and void such traditional distinctions and the ethical guidelines that controlled them.

Are we therefore delivered up—bound hand and foot—to the supposedly therapeutic determination of a constantly expanding techno-medical power? Demands for the right to die and to die with dignity oppose that power.

And this brings us back to the question of the meaning and mastery of life. Who is master of my life? Who, if not I, can determine its meaning? What determines for me—for others and ultimately for all humankind—the quality of life and of the death that terminates it?

IKEDA • In 1991, a Japanese doctor administered a fatal injection of potassium chloride to a terminally ill patient and was accused of murder. Failing to ascertain the patient's wishes, he acted on the basis of a request from family members. What he did cannot exactly be called euthanasia, but it is likely that in the future, as an increasing number of patients request euthanasia, actions like his will be repeated.

BOURGEAULT • The debate on euthanasia is colored by a plurality of views and opinions on life and its human quality. Some people advocate complete and absolute respect for human life out of belief in its sanctity. Others demand that individual personal decisions and judgments about the quality of life be taken into consideration. Some of the latter feel life is no longer worth living when we can no longer maintain and improve its quality—that at this point, it is not worth or no longer worth living. Though one cannot take the life of another (against that person's will or without that person's stated volition), it should at least be possible to terminate life for oneself. Respect for life can thus legitimate deliberate action for its termination. This is where euthanasia comes in.

If the principle of the sanctity of life is contested, can we define rules of conduct that, if not eliminating all risk, at least prevent abuse? Ethical guidelines on respect for life and its human quality in the relativist, pluralist context I have already mentioned have been put forth. I am thinking, for instance, of advances made over the past decade by the Canadian Law Reform Commission that define the appropriate legal framework for cessation of treatment and euthanasia. The guidelines favor life, respect for personal autonomy, and the individual right to self-determination. They specifically take quality of life and protection of the weakest members of society into consideration.

IKEDA · In the court ruling on the 1991 murder case I mentioned earlier, active euthanasia was deemed permissible in Japan under the following conditions: unbearable physical pain; inevitability and imminence of death; exhaustion of known methods for eliminating or alleviating physical pain and lack of alternatives; and clear indication of the patient's consent to having life shortened.

In the West, the lower house of the Dutch parliament recently adopted guidelines on euthanasia after years of debate.

BOURGEAULT · The November 2000 adoption of euthanasia legislation by the Netherlands Parliament has certainly not closed the discussion. But the polemics leading up to it were highly educational. They serve as a kind of summation of the developments of the last decade. What is sometimes called the Dutch model is not without interest. The code of conduct governing medical practice in the matter of euthanasia in Holland is summarized in the following three general requirements. (1) After obligatory consultation with other physicians, the doctor in charge must establish that the seriousness of the patient's condition precludes hope and submit this conclusion to the hospital administration. (2) The doctor must inform the patient of the gravity of the condition and of foreseeable developments, which will determine the orientation of subsequent care. (3) The doctor must receive formal, express, and repeated requests from the patient in question for euthanasia. To keep both patient and colleague-consultants well informed, the doctor must keep a logbook recording details of the treatment and the consecutive reactions of the patient.

These rules generally satisfy the demands of prudence and vigilance. They call for circumspection on the part of the doctor, and for supervision of the medical treatment by the patient, colleagues, and the administration of the institution. They demand vigilance from everyone. The requirement of a log or medical file and of disclosure and consultation forbids all precipitate action. The patient must make a "current" explicit request (expressing a decision taken in the currently experienced situation) and repeat it. Since a "living will" drawn up beforehand is considered invalid, this would seem to exclude recourse to euthanasia on the request of another person when the patient cannot express his or her will.

As debates surrounding the adoption of the law in November 2000 indicated, however, things are not actually that clear. While many Dutch citizens now carry what is called a "euthanasia passport," we are witnessing an upsurge of anti-euthanasia sentiment. On principle or out of conviction, and sometimes out of fear of abuse, more than 20,000 people carry what they call "life passports." Nor does their fear seem irrational. Results of studies made before and after the adoption of these new practices show that, in spite of regulations, in the past few years, more than a thousand cases of non-voluntary euthanasia were performed annually.

IKEDA • Recent discussions on active euthanasia in Europe and North America emphasize the patient's right to self-determination and seem to be moving in the direction of allowing euthanasia when the will of the patient can be ascertained.

Nonetheless, Buddhists are fundamentally against any form of assisted death. The progress of medical treatment—including methods used in palliative care units—offers hope, even though treatment cannot totally eliminate suffering. Still, instead of taking this as a reason to affirm active euthanasia, the Buddhist preference is to seek to support methods of alleviating unbearable pain through medical advances and the care provided by family, friends and the medical team.

Buddhism teaches that human life is invaluable, because Buddha nature is inherent in every person. Assisted death may deprive someone of the possibility of manifesting Buddha nature. This is why we must oppose euthanasia.

BOURGEAULT • I can understand the Buddhist way of thinking quite well.

Ethical guidelines and rules for euthanasia

IKEDA • Since the 1970s, developments in euthanasia-related discussions in the United States have led to a radical change in direction. Former emphasis on easing suffering has recently shifted to "death with dignity." In cases of incurable illness, as the end draws near, people wish to maintain their pride, self-respect, and some control over their faculties and personal dignity. One of the reasons for the change in emphasis is certainly growing awareness of patients' rights, including the right to die. Without the possibilities offered to us today by medical science, this right would be purely theoretical.

Medical science has made great progress in the development of treatments that relieve pain and eliminate the agony of illness. Sophisticated technology has developed support equipment to greatly prolong life. The down side of these advances, however, is that they at times maintain patients in vegetative states, from whence the moral question: Does a comatose or nearly comatose patient with no hope of recovery, plugged into an artificial respirator and attached to feeding tubes and various other machines, possess true human dignity?

BOURGEAULT • Doctors in Quebec—as in France, Switzerland, and surely elsewhere—insist on a distinction between euthanasia and what we call "total sedation" to relieve patient suffering. According to some, this distinction sets up a tenuous, practically imperceptible, even nonexistent border because both total sedation and euthanasia entail irreversible loss of consciousness.

Sedation or euthanasia? In either case, ethical guidelines must be proposed and rules of conduct enforced to counter possible abuses of people who may be kept almost indefinitely in a degenerative state.

IKEDA • I agree. Dying with dignity is an integral part of the responsibility of each individual as a human being. Human life is dignified in and of itself, as is every patient and every family, not to mention the doctor-patient relationship, which is based on mutual respect. Today, however, it is extremely difficult to maintain that dignity in relationships dominated by therapeutic technologies that far outstrip advances in medical ethics. It is of vital importance to carefully examine all the issues surrounding the dignified death of people in a vegetative condition.

BOURGEAULT • I only learned of my teacher Professor Laperrière's death several years after the fact, so I have no idea how he died. But when I saw Professor Labelle, after I had begun teaching, he was seriously ill. Despite his illness, he was still interested in everyone around him. Amazingly, he preserved the enthusiasm of his younger years. Although he knew he would not live much longer, he never mentioned it and was not depressed. He devoted himself to helping others. Seeing him do it moved me deeply.

Maintaining the creative capacity to serve others

IKEDA • That brings to mind the last hours of Shakyamuni, who announced his own death three months before it happened. Just before the end, a monk by the name of Subhadda came to see him, but a disciple named Ananda intercepted him, saying that Shakyamuni was too tired to be disturbed. Subhadda came three times. On the last occasion, hearing of his arrival, Shakyamuni received him and earnestly related how, ever since abandoning the secular world, he had always walked in the way of justice and the Law. Subhadda became Shakyamuni's last disciple. He later said, "The Revered One revealed the truth in many ways as if he were lighting lamps in the dark." As this episode reveals, by expounding the Law for the sake of saving humanity until the final days of his life, Shakyamuni showed his disciples how to die with human dignity.

My mentor, Josei Toda, died with dignity. From his sickbed, he encouraged others and answered questions about Buddhism. Until his last breath, he gave advice to people in distress. All his life, he radiated health in the true sense of the word, even after he became ill.

BOURGEAULT • My mentor, Mr. Cormier, was a champion of human rights who maintained his dignity, too. "I'm not sick. It is just my body that is being attacked by cancer." He fulfilled the definition of health as something a person can deal with physically, psychologically, economically, socially and culturally. He never regarded his cancer as a "sickness" but as a condition he could continue to cope with in the above ways.

IKEDA • True health does not mean the absence of illness. Rather, it is a life-state characterized by openness to the hearts and minds of others and to the environment. It is constant readiness to exercise the creative ability to serve society. To maintain health in that sense until the last moment is to die with dignity.

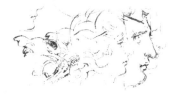

5. Confronting Death

Quality instead of quantity

IKEDA • Advances in modern medicine greatly prolong the pre-death period, giving patients in the terminal phase of their illness much more time to live in the face of death. Consequently, one of the main concerns of contemporary medicine is to find ways to support the dying so they can overcome fear and anxiety. This is why terminal care has become a focus of great attention.

BOURGEAULT • During the past twenty years, a number of hospices have been established in Canada. I am familiar only with those in Montreal and Quebec. They give good service but are too few in number, which makes their patients seem privileged. Some people, however, reject reliance on such specialized institutions, preferring to keep patients at home as long as possible, sometimes right up until death, providing all the medical and paramedical support needed—especially pain relief.

IKEDA • Of course, hospices are not the only solution for terminal care. Palliative home care is also very important. Whether at home or elsewhere, we expect palliative care to encourage a religious or spiritual attitude in the face of death, to help patients deal with the end of their lives and to go beyond the attitudes of modern civilization, which present death in a very negative light. Indeed, determining existential issues such as how a person should live out the final chapter of life is exactly the kind of question religion is expected to answer.

BOURGEAULT • I consider it necessary to encourage and sustain in practical terms all efforts to make life worthwhile and dignified to the end. I think I have already mentioned Trémolières's words to the effect that it is better to add life to years than to add years to life. Life expectancy today is increasing. We must interpret the increase more qualitatively than quantitatively.

IKEDA • Precisely. Spiritual considerations have incited people to look much more closely at institutionalized care. Institutions are designed to provide the necessary personnel: doctors, nurses, social workers, aids, and volunteers, and often religious counselors or clergy as well. The goal is to allow the patient to live as fully as possible by providing spiritual support, for the patient as well as the family. The hospice is not just a place to prepare for death but also the last place one lives, and where one rounds out one's life.

Elisabeth Kübler-Ross (1926–) speaks of a five-stage process the patient undergoes upon realizing that death is drawing near. The first is denial, followed by anger at fate. In the third stage, the patient bargains with supernatural beings like God or the Buddha. If nothing results from the bargaining, the next stage is depression, followed by acceptance.

At the approach of death, the mind of the patient is heavy with anger, sadness and depression. It is the role of the terminal-caregiver to help the patient adopt a positive approach, overcome the suffering of death, and make the fullest, most self-expressive use of the remaining time. This role will be of growing significance in the years to come.

BOURGEAULT · Yes, but that said, I distrust—and I am not alone in this—the current tendency to sweeten death. You mention the ideas and work of Elisabeth Kübler-Ross. On the basis of innumerable dialogues with hospitalized dying patients, she presents death as a reality to be accepted and experienced as the final stage of growth. The acceptance is preceded by sometimes aggressive denial.[3]

The testimonies she reports are often touching. They come from dying people who, informed of the gravity of their illnesses, find themselves obliged to prepare for death. Although they remain clear-minded, their failing powers seemingly facilitate a relinquishment—or in Kübler-Ross's term, letting go—that is as much biological and physical as psychological and spiritual. They are accompanied in their illness by relatives, sometimes friends, members of the medical-care team, and by either Kübler-Ross herself or people who share her philosophy or spirituality.

IKEDA · Buddhism establishes three categories of pain: physical; psychological—caused by loss; and existential—caused by awareness of

3. Elisabeth Kübler-Ross. *On Death and Dying.* New York: MacMillan. 1969. *Death: The Final Stage.* New York: MacMillan. 1975.

the transitory nature of the phenomenal world. Death and the fear of death are said to be the conjunction of these three.

The first type of pain can be alleviated with the help of medical science. Social welfare systems and the combined cooperative efforts of family and the medical system can lighten psychological suffering. Overcoming existential suffering, however, is another story altogether. This is the anguish caused by the idea of our own mortality. I am convinced that a way of thinking about life and death and of triumphing over the fear and apprehension of death rooted in eternal truths is necessary. If people can internalize a spiritual view of life and death, it will enable them to overcome the despair of these three types of pain and greet the final chapter of their lives, tranquil and fulfilled.

BOURGEAULT • But very large numbers of people die abandoned or the victims of epidemics, famine, accidents, catastrophes, or war, often without regaining consciousness. All of these people who die violently and alone—and they are probably in the majority—fall outside the Kübler-Ross experience, limiting, though not invalidating, its pertinence.

Near-death experiences

IKEDA • That is very true. Still, many people have described near-death experiences. Sometimes when accidents, illness, or surgery leave people in a state of lowered consciousness and bring them to the point where death is actually encountered, these people regain consciousness—or "come back to life"—and relate their experiences.

Since 1975, when the American internist Raymond A. Moody, Jr. (1944–) published *Life after Life: The Investigation of a Phenomenon, Survival of Bodily Death*, many physicians, psychologists, and psychiatrists have published data on the same phenomenon.

Dr. Moody derived the following basic patterns from the experiences he collected. The most commonly experienced phenomena include the sensation of passing through a long tunnel just when the doctor pronounces the subject dead, followed by sudden consciousness of separation from the physical body, encounters with others, recollections of major life events, and the appearance of life as light. Later research has shown that these patterns are generally shared.

BOURGEAULT • Moody's book was a best seller in Canada, as elsewhere. It seems to me that the phenomena he lists can be explained differently and more simply than he suggests. Perhaps I am over-rationalizing—maybe that is a habit of my job. You yourself refer to psychology. The knowledge we have of the physiological and psychological mechanisms of perception explains the phenomena in question in a way that, though nuanced and fragile, satisfies me better than the way proposed by Moody and his colleagues—or disciples.

Several years ago, the theologian and psychoanalyst, Louis Beirnaert (1906–85) compared the mystical visions of Saint Ignatius de Loyola (1419?–1556) with those of prisoners of the Dachau concentration camp. He explained the similarities he observed as resulting from rigorous fasting, voluntary on the one hand and harshly imposed on the other. He added that the mystical saint probably experienced changes in body chemistry identical with those experienced by the starving prisoners and that these changes no doubt accounted for the similarity of their so-called visions. Saint Ignatius gave his own visions—or hallucinations—a different significance. It seems to me that the exhaustion of vital resources could account for Moody's observations.

IKEDA • Near-death experiences are frequently analyzed and interpreted as psychological phenomena, like drug-induced hallucinations, paroxysms of the temporal lobe, or cerebral disorders resulting from oxygen deprivation. As a Buddhist, I hope that much more data on near-death experiences will be gathered and analyzed from the perspectives of psychology, physiology, psychopathology, ethnology, and anthropology.

BOURGEAULT • Nonetheless, I must admit that I am uneasy whenever the meaninglessness of death—and the radical rupture it causes—seems to be denied by affirmations of continuity of life and some kind of survival assured by its renewal. This appears to me to be consolation-seeking—the legitimacy of which, in spite of everything, I recognize.

No matter what is said, death marks a radical rupture. The prospect of death confronts the living person, who has given meaning to and sought to enjoy life, with an absurd alternative. On the one hand, survival that, in spite of the most intense desire, cannot succeed in truly saving life and whatever gives it richness, savor, and value. On the other hand, annihilation reducing everything to inconceivable oblivion.

Facing death boldly

IKEDA • Montaigne said, "To philosophize is to learn to die."[4] Similarly, Buddhism teaches us: "First learn about death, and then about other matters."[5] As both statements suggest, learning about death enriches life.

No matter how we interpret near-death experiences, the lives of people who have undergone them have been revolutionized. Some have reported that a face-to-face encounter with death caused them to reflect critically on the way they had been living and to try to live as fully as possible, so as to be prepared for death whenever it might come.

I think you will agree with me on the following points: First, people who have undergone near-death experiences no longer fear dying. Second, as long as they go on living, they strive to acquire knowledge. Third, no longer egotistically concerned with fame, power, and wealth, they resolve to live altruistically and compassion-ately. If we can return from death's doorstep with this kind of change in attitude, then I believe such an experience is very valuable for whoever experiences it.

In my 1993 speech at Harvard, on Mahayana Buddhism and Twenty-First Century Civilization, I pointed out that people today have averted their eyes from the problem of dying and given it a negative image diametrically opposed to the positive image of living. I called for people to bravely face death instead of ignoring it.

BOURGEAULT • In Canada and generally in North America, it has become extremely difficult to accept the negative aspects of the evolution of

---

4. *The Complete Essays of Montaigne.* Tr. Donald M. Frame. Stanford, CA: Stanford University Press. 1958.
5. *Gosho Zenshu.* 1404.

life for what they are. This can be attributed to the idea that when life encounters death, it can no longer expand but is condemned to the ultimate stage, that of extinction.

IKEDA • Buddhism is based on the principle of *hossho no kimetsu* or the manifestation and latency of the eternal truth inherent in all things. According to this principle, *hossho*[6] or that which is eternally true, becomes manifest and latent repeatedly in accordance with its karmic relationships with all phenomena—including life and death—and this process accounts for the creative quality of evolution.

BOURGEAULT • Can life, defined and constantly compelled by creative personal liberty, escape death? Jean-Paul Sartre (1905–80) and Simone de Beauvoir (1908–86), both non-believers and atheists, ascribed to a view and a dynamic that defy death and its meaninglessness and seek to break its hold on life. In a sense, through the soaring of the thoughts that constitute our humanity and give meaning to our lives, through the bonds of love and friendship, through our children, and through the works we leave behind us, we each transcend the death that will ultimately engulf us. Because death is stronger than we are, and its meaninglessness drives us up against the absurd, even during life. But does death swallow everything up? Beyond death there remains what Jean-Paul Sartre called being-for-others. The French philosopher Vladimir Jankélévitch (1903–85) would also evoke the "having been," "having lived," and "having loved."

IKEDA • I agree with Sartre and Jankélévitch on that point. Life is short and what we can accomplish during its brief duration is naturally limited. Nonetheless, those who come after us as heirs to our achievements, and those who are influenced by what we have done, give our lives immortality.

Worldwide SGI anti-war, pro-peace, and pro–human-well-being activities are founded on Josei Toda's heritage, expressed most notably

6. One of the most fundamental concepts of Buddhism, *hossho* has many different meanings. It is most often used to mean: (1) the Law, or ultimate truth; (2) the teaching of the Buddha who reveals the Law, or sutras; (3) the manifestations of the Law—phenomena, things, facts, existences, etc.; (4) the aspects of existence which, according to the Theravada school, are the most fundamental components of the individual and his or her reality; and (5) the precepts or behavior that leads to the accumulation of good karma.

in his condemnation of nuclear weapons and his philosophy of global citizenship. As our activities spread around the world, we have the firm conviction that our first president Tsunesaburo Makiguchi and Mr. Toda "live" today in SGI members and all our undertakings.

6. Birth

IKEDA • Buddhism emphasizes the equal importance of birth and death by combining the words in a single compound term, *shoji.*

BOURGEAULT • Birth is as decisive for humans as death. And the moment at which human life starts is just as hard to determine as the moment when it ends.

IKEDA • What are the Christian views of this topic?

BOURGEAULT • In the Judeo-Christian tradition, life was described in such terms as *psyche* (soul; literally, breath) and *pneuma* (vital spirit; literally, wind). This corresponds to the ancient belief that life is animated by some substance flowing inside the body. People believed that life came from the Spirit of God and therefore had to be treated with the greatest care and respect.

Later, after Christianity was established, imposed Christian civilization and adopted the Greco-Roman heritage, discussions about life took a different turn. For instance, attention was directed toward determining the moment when life becomes human, the moment in its development when the fetus becomes a human entity.

IKEDA • In other words, emphasis shifted from the appearance of life to the birth of the human being.

BOURGEAULT • Yes. People tried to distinguish between the embryo and the completed human being. Paradoxically, some people came up with the discriminatory thesis that a male fetus becomes human after three months' pregnancy but that this occurs only after six months' pregnancy in the case of a female fetus. The traditional view that the fetus becomes human when it starts breathing by itself—that is, at birth—finally held sway.

Recently people have been using the completely unscientific term *pre-embryos* to designate so-called young embryos frozen for implantation or for research purposes. Actually, I think it is impossible to determine the precise moment when human life begins or actually becomes human. The process is perhaps gradual in that, with the passing time, the human entity grows in complexity until it finally becomes human.

IKEDA • Buddhist scriptures hold that life begins at the moment of conception. Modern prenatal physiology clearly reveals conditions in the mother's womb that were impossible to determine in ancient times. To deal with the issues of in vitro fertilization and artificial insemination, we must re-examine our interpretation of the nature of life on the basis of scientific and medical findings.

Buddhism teaches that birth, like death, is a process. Some sutras describe conception as the establishment of an "entity of intermediary existence" or the introduction of consciousness. The consciousness in question here is the eighth or *alaya* consciousness, the collective subconscious I mentioned earlier in relation to death. From the viewpoint of reincarnation, life is an "intermediary existence" between the moment of death and the moment of the next birth. Conception is the moment when this intermediary existence is wedded to its next human form. As the embryo develops, the other levels of consciousness develop: first the seventh, then the mind or sixth consciousness, and finally the five senses.

Cerebral physiology divides fetal development into two stages. During the initial five to six months of pregnancy, cell division, proliferation, and movement take place. During the second stage, networking functions evolve—neurites, axones, dendrites and synapses develop. The second stage is a process during which the various functions of the human body emerge. Scientific discoveries seem to confirm the Buddhist interpretation in which the subconscious, the conscious and the five senses gradually emerge.

This concept of birth as a process agrees with your theory of the increasing complexity of the developing human entity.

Ethical issues in prenatal diagnosis

IKEDA • Recent technological progress has been made at a dizzying speed. It is not surprising that technology, which makes artificial manipulation of human life possible, is generating new and serious ethical problems.

The possibility of prenatal examinations has added new aspects to the issue of artificially induced abortion. Prenatal tests like amniocentesis, ultrasound, and chorionic villi sampling (cvs) allow us to monitor the very early stages of fetal development and identify a growing number of congenital and hereditary disorders.

BOURGEAULT • In effect, well before birth, prenatal tests—pre-implantation tests in the case of in vitro fertilization—reveal the "quality" of life in store for the gestating human being if it is allowed to develop. New options present new questions. The need to choose among them continues to the end of life. In its very last moments, we can partially dissociate life from suffering and agony. We are in a position to hasten or retard death itself, whose ancient power can be, if not abolished, perhaps held temporarily in check.

IKEDA • Apparently the maternal serum marker test (or maternal serological screening) is very easy to perform. This test could easily be included as a standard prenatal test without debating its ethical implications. To examine this and other similar problems, the Japanese Ministry of Health and Welfare set up a committee of specialists, in October 1998, to deliberate ethical issues and the safety of prenatal diagnoses, including pre-implantation diagnoses. Where does Canadian medical opinion stand on this issue?

BOURGEAULT • A 1990 inquiry at twenty-two specialized centers in Canada revealed that frequent recourse to prenatal diagnosis is becoming practically routine. It is part of the usual prevention protocol or follow-up for pregnant women over 35 years old or women who have reason to fear giving birth to a malformed child or a child with a grave hereditary sickness.[7] In 1990, of the at least 22,000 women who visited one or another of these 22 centers, 78% did so because of age (older than 35 during pregnancy). The others had

7. Based on research reports conducted under the auspices of the Royal Commission on New Reproductive Technologies led by Dr. Patricia A. Baird, and specifically on Volumes 12 and 13 on prenatal diagnosis in Canada, annexed to the official report entitled *Proceed With Care.*

various reasons such as previous personal experiences, family history, or abnormal results from routine examinations.

Generally the women interviewed considered prenatal diagnostic tests useful, if unpleasant. They were universally satisfied with services offered or actually rendered. But—before, during, and after the tests and possible subsequent treatments—they wished that the overall process was managed in such a way that their actual experiences were taken into account. The doctors and "genetic counselors" were on the whole favorable to general implementation of these tests for women over 35 and for women with some reason to fear giving birth to an infant suffering from an anomaly or a serious condition. There was also a fairly broad consensus on the need to communicate the results of the tests to the women, so they could freely give informed consent to continue or terminate their pregnancy.

IKEDA · If a congenital deformation is detected, the decision of whether to carry the child to term is left to the mother. The burden of the child's abnormality falls on one woman's shoulders, when it ought to rest with society as a whole.

BOURGEAULT · Can such a thing be called freedom? In another Canadian inquiry—this one, too, conducted in 1990—the women interviewed generally affirmed that their freedom to choose had been respected. Several indicated, however, that a subtle pressure was exerted on them, arising more from a prevailing atmosphere or the general influence of a dominant ideology than from a particular professional's desire to impose his or her viewpoint.

The women felt and lived an ambivalence related to two social constructs or two images of pregnancy—on the one hand, a rich, natural experience affecting their entire being, and on the other, reduction to the object of tests performed with the help of diverse techniques and analyses. The book *Women's Experience with Technology in Pregnancy*, written by Sari Tidiver at about the time of this survey, looks closely at this ambivalence. It casts in sharp relief the limits that various pressures impose on women's liberty. It also explores the women's dissatisfaction at seeing their experiences ignored in a process fragmented into a series of separate medical procedures.

Many women who underwent prenatal diagnoses expressed ambiguous or ambivalent feelings and sometimes resentment. They realized that the technology had simultaneously helped and invaded them, and that afterward they were left on their own to make difficult decisions. Here we have a double paradox. Since the child is wanted, pregnancy itself is often wanted and experienced as a happy event. This rich and fulfilling experience is suddenly troubled and tormented by the possibility—suggested by the very proposal to undergo prenatal diagnosis—of an "abnormal" birth. Yet the proposed tests are a reasonable and necessary outcropping of the mother's sense of responsibility to her unborn infant. When the results are bad, however, the technological equipment believed to make possible the birth of a perfect baby fails, abandoning the woman to her sadness and distress.

IKEDA • If the kind of responsibility you have just described is imposed on pregnant women, prenatal diagnosis is more likely to curtail than to strengthen their rights. Society already exerts many pressures on women—both implicitly and explicitly—especially in the areas of giving birth and raising children. Providing equipment for prenatal testing is important, but we must also create the kind of social system that can support and advise women trapped in untenable situations.

BOURGEAULT • In certain cases, prenatal diagnosis permits us to detect anomalies or pathological conditions. But the genetic therapies that will someday effect the necessary corrections are not ready, at least not in the majority of cases. In practice, the objective of prenatal diagnosis is usually information—forecasts or "predictions"—and "prevention" in the form of pregnancy termination.

IKEDA • In Japan, when amniotic-fluid tests reveal fetal anomalies, abortion is considered as a matter of course. This is one of the major problems with prenatal tests.

Quality of life

BOURGEAULT • Here we encounter the crucial and fundamental questions of bioethics. What do we mean by genetic anomaly? What is susceptibility or predisposition to such-and-such a sickness? What is abnormality? What is a handicap? At what stage can we judge these ills serious enough to justify abortion?

Two questions among the many capture the attention. First is the definition of the boundary between normal and abnormal (or pathological). To establish this boundary is to define the quality of human life. The second question, underlying the first, deals with so-called soft eugenics.

IKEDA · Both truly fundamental questions.

BOURGEAULT · The definition of the quality of life harks back to the concepts of normal and pathological. Some sufferers from serious, genetically transmitted defects or diseases consider their lives happy and worth living. Contrary to our spontaneous judgments and the opinion of specialists, they believe their lives have truly human quality.

Essentially, a handicap is not so much a medical problem as a social problem, a matter of social acceptance. In any case, who can judge the quality of life of a person as yet unborn? Drawing boundaries between the normal and the pathological is not easy.

IKEDA · I agree entirely. In March and June 1998, the Japan Society of Obstetrics and Gynecology sponsored public discussion meetings of pre-implantation diagnosis. A representative of the disabled spoke at the meetings, insisting above all that the presence of disabled people in the world should be considered a given, that we must eliminate all discrimination against them and instead offer them all the support they need to take their rightful place in society.

In defining quality of life, we must not draw boundaries and relegate everything beyond those boundaries to the "abnormal." Instead we must do everything in our power to build the kind of broadminded society in which people living with disabilities do not have to consider themselves "handicapped" and can manifest their full potential.

BOURGEAULT · Testimonials received in numerous inquiries demonstrate remarkably unanimous rejection of the use of prenatal diagnostics for eugenic ends. Nonetheless, all genetic research, intervention, and medicine seem to me to fall into the category of what I call soft eugenics. Throughout life and even before birth, we attempt to improve the health of individuals and whole populations, not by suppressing handicaps—as has been done in many countries, not only in Nazi Germany during the thirties—not by what I call hard eugenics, but by soft eugenics. Soft eugenics begins before birth, in the egg, if I may put it that way.

IKEDA • People are often suspicious of eugenics because of its link with Nazi policies of racism and ethnic cleansing.

BOURGEAULT • In my opinion, we must tackle the ethical debate on eugenics on new grounds. If we believe that life is not simply handed to us as a divine gift but is entrusted to our responsibility, we cannot condemn all forms of eugenics out of hand and a priori.

IKEDA • Of course, everyone wishes to have healthy children. If reproductive technologies can help, their use should be considered with all necessary prudence. But I am apprehensive that this might lead to interventions unfavorable to life itself. Though the object of reproductive technologies is the fetus, society or individuals might use these technologies to control or impose constraints on the lives of others. In keeping with the Buddhist concept of the sacredness of life, we must demonstrate extreme caution in applying technologies capable of manipulating life itself.

We must also take into consideration effects on the mother's body of carrying the child to term. All decisions must be made carefully and with the cooperation of both parents and the medical team to find the solution that is most beneficial to the child.

Abortion and a feminine philosophy of life

IKEDA • I understand that you participated in discussions on bioethics concerning abortion in Canada.

BOURGEAULT • During the tumultuous debates held in Quebec at the beginning of the 1970s on decriminalizing abortion, I helped write a report for the League of Human Rights (later renamed the League of Rights and Liberties). The title of the report discreetly indicates its fundamental orientation: *Quebec Society Facing Abortion.*[8]

Discussions and legislation against abortion are often hypocritical. As is clearly evident in the United States, those who condemn

---

8. *La société québécoise face à l'avortement.* Montréal: Leméac. 1973. The French expression "face à" has a connotation of opposition.

abortion—more often men than women—call for the maintenance or restoration of the death penalty, defend the right to possess and use arms, and favor repression of criminals and deviants over social aid and reform. This stance is full of contradictions: the right to life is blindly defended on the one hand and summarily denied on the other. Moreover, what ought to be a shared responsibility is unloaded on women.

Abortion is connected with social issues. Poverty and its consequences frequently thwart the possibility of even carrying pregnancy to term (in Quebec and the rest of Canada, single mothers are among the poorest of the poor). Job insecurity is another key factor: the free play of competition—itself a cause of unemployment—threatens rights we thought were ensured, like maternity leave. Then there is inadequate community support: both the government and the church display an indifference that belies their words.

Our report recalled the responsibility of society—that is, of each of its members. Participants in the working group unanimously agreed that it is absurd to separate the right to life and the right to freedom. Respect for life and respect for rights and freedoms are inseparable. Respect for life has no meaning if that life is not free. But the converse also is true: rights and freedoms are impossible without respect for life.

IKEDA • What you say is very wise. I too feel that the concept of respect for life and the insistence on rights and freedoms can be made compatible. Unfortunately, in Japan, with little public discussion, abortion is used as a means of population control. In consequence, reproductive technology tends to be seen as a mere medical treatment. The ethics of the issue go largely unconsidered, and legal restrictions are lax.

BOURGEAULT • The women I have met over the years have seemed very solicitous of life. They have equally rejected the intransigence of grand principles and rules on the one hand, and judgments and condemnations on the other. They have made me examine my own personal rapport with life—with my own life and with the lives of others.

We must remember, however, that termination of pregnancy is not the only solution to problems occasionally revealed by prenatal diagnosis. In certain cases, gene therapy is now effective. Hopes aroused by treatments still in their infancy will surely not all be deceived.[9]

IKEDA • While women are obviously the most profoundly affected by it, abortion is intimately entwined with the attitudes the mother, both parents, the family and society at large hold toward the fetus. The issue requires serious, considered debate.

Buddhist compassion extends to respect for fetal life. It prefers avoiding abortion in favor of other methods of contraception.

Of course, other considerations play a role. When birth endangers the mother's life or when pregnancy is the result of rape or other violent sexual relations, the will of the parents—especially the mother—must be respected in making a decision.

If genetic therapy progresses far enough in the future and provides solutions for certain problems, it should be considered as an option, but first it must be carefully and seriously examined to determine the best way to use it. Of course, all possible precautions must be taken to prevent therapy from degenerating into the manipulation of people for non-therapeutic ends.

I believe that traditionally, Christianity—particularly Catholicism—has forbidden abortion out of respect for life as a gift from God.

BOURGEAULT • I have two comments to make on that topic. First, there is no clear reference to abortion in the Bible. Second, there is an obvious contradiction between the logic of the Crusades and the so-called just wars, of the Inquisition and religious torture, capital punishment and so on—a logic, long embraced by Christianity, that excludes all dissidents and denies their right to life—and the permanent interdiction of abortion on the basis of respect for the dignity of human life.

IKEDA • Buddhism is founded on tolerance. Just as the Buddhist precept against taking life extends to fetal life, this spirit of toleration recognizes the dignity of all life. This logic of tolerance could provide the foundation for a society that values individuality and enables people to live in self-respect, confident of the future. Modern society as a whole must effect a shift from the logic of exclusion to the logic of tolerance, which makes harmonious coexistence possible.

9. Based on *Proceed With Care,* the report published in 1993 by the Royal Commission on New Reproductive Technologies, led by Dr. Patricia A. Baird.

7. Reproductive Technology

Abuse of reproductive technology

IKEDA • The use of biotechnology based on emerging life sciences now permits such life-manipulative technologies as artificial insemination, in vitro fertilization, and embryo transplants.

BOURGEAULT • Thanks to scientific and technological developments, we can now give substance to our dreams. As Jean-François Malherbe remarked in discussing the ethical aspects of medically assisted procreation, three ancient dreams have now been realized.[10] First, thanks to various contraceptive techniques, it is possible to avoid having unwanted children. Second, even sterile people can have children by way of artificial insemination, in vitro fertilization, and surrogacy. And third, thanks to prenatal diagnosis, abortion and, soon, genetic intervention, it is possible to have only the kind of children one wants.

IKEDA • How are such life-manipulative techniques evaluated in Canada from the bioethical standpoint? How do Canadians feel they can be used to benefit humanity?

BOURGEAULT • Between 1990 and 1993, the debate on these issues was nourished by the work and frank discussions of the Royal Commission on New Reproductive Technologies. In addition to its report, in 1993, this commission published fifteen lengthy supplements detailing the results of its inquiries and research.

In the wake of these consultations, the Canadian parliament began work on a bill to control new reproductive technologies and eliminate all kinds of commercialization and possible irregularities. The measures in the bill were intended to forbid certain practices current in the United States and elsewhere—sometimes even in Canada. For instance, recourse to surrogacy, selection of fetus sex for non-medical reasons, trafficking in ova and sperm cells (only unremunerated donations are permitted), sales and purchase of embryos, development of embryos in artificial uteruses, cloning of human embryos,

---

10. Édouard Boné and Jean-François Malherbe. *Engendrés par la science: enjeux éthiques des manipulations de la procréation* (Engendered by Science: The Ethical Issues of Reproductive Technology). Paris: Éditions du Cerf. 1985.

creation of human/animal hybrids, transfer of human embryos into animals, development and conservation of human embryos for research purposes, and sampling ova or sperm from cadavers.

Some of the measures announced were generally well received. Others aroused reservations and outright opposition from people who felt that they would only nourish unfounded apprehensions. To use the time-honored expression, the bill died on the Order Paper. A second bill met the same fate.

Louise Vandelac, a sociologist with a lively interest in these questions, lamented that after a $30 million commission and two bills killed before they saw the light of day, Canada still has not defined a specific legal framework for such matters. The medical technology industry prospers with little or no regulation. Still, the debate goes on.

IKEDA • Artificial insemination is currently practiced in many countries. Homologous insemination—artificial insemination by the husband—has proven to be an effective procedure in infertility cases and provokes few problems, since the child is genetically the couple's, however much medical technology may have contributed to its birth. On the other hand, when sperm is provided by a donor—heterologous insemination—serious bioethical problems may arise, even though the technology is the same.

In America, reproductive functions are already being commercialized. Some sperm banks collect the sperm of celebrated people like Nobel Prize laureates and Olympic athletes, and agencies can be hired to find surrogate mothers and oversee the birth and placement of the child. I am opposed to the practice of selecting certain types of sperm for artificial insemination. The dignity of human life does not depend on IQ or special abilities. It is determined by the kind of life a person lives.

Fundamental human rights have been infringed in connection with the commercialization of reproductive technology. One court case closely followed by the media concerned the bitter battle of a divorced couple over frozen fertilized ova. In another case, a surrogate mother who had grown attached to the child she was carrying decided to keep him, provoking a heart-rending legal battle with the woman who had hired her. In an even more tragic case, a baby born through surrogacy had a congenital abnormality and the contracting couple refused to "take delivery."

Disintegration or transformation of the family

BOURGEAULT • Today we dissociate procreation from formerly indispensable sexual relations and from traditional forms of paternity and maternity. As you have noted, this dissociation is not without risk. By opening the door to new relationships, it forces us to re-evaluate the connections between emotional life, sexual relations and commitment, in individual lives, in the framework of social relations, and in the reconstitution of what we call the family, which has taken so many forms throughout time and from civilization to civilization. It also entails the risk of the abuses you have already underscored: commercialization of human life; blatant or concealed eugenics; hopes betrayed; disillusionment; judicial battles in which individuals—children above all—pay the price, since their rights are trampled; and— lest we forget—the possibility of sorcerer's apprentices in the form of inept practitioners.

IKEDA • Before turning to reproductive technologies, would-be parents must first address such basic questions as why they want a child and what they are prepared to do for the child. If parents can overcome their egotism and feel joy and gratitude at helping their child live a life worthy of humanity, the disintegration of the family can be avoided. It would then be possible to build the family on the basis of the new relationships you mention.

Since its first successful performance in England in 1978, in vitro fertilization has become everyday technology all over the world.

BOURGEAULT • Experimental and innovative research and practices in the field of assisted procreation are generally carried out in university centers, where regular exchanges among researchers and practitioners on the one hand and various evaluation and control mechanisms on the other at least limit the risks, even if they can never be totally eliminated. We can feel generally confident but we must remain vigilant, especially in the face of the proliferation of private research and treatment centers. In my opinion, a responsible ethic requires us not to reject innovation but to limit its risks and curtail, if possible, its harmful effects ahead of time.

IKEDA • No medical treatment is without risk. Reproductive technologies are no exception. Absolute priority must be given to ethical considerations and to the safety of individuals. This responsibility falls largely to the professionals who engage in this rapidly evolving field.

In the final analysis, the parents' responsibility toward a child born with the help of medical technology must dictate the use of that technology. Parents who care for their children must cautiously approach the use of reproductive technology on the foundation of firm views on life—how they themselves live and the kind of life they want for their child.

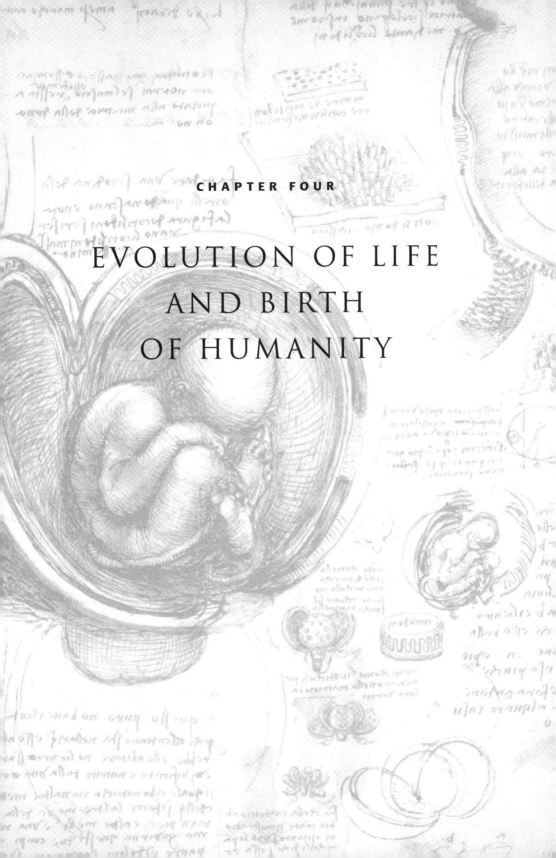

CHAPTER FOUR

EVOLUTION OF LIFE
AND BIRTH
OF HUMANITY

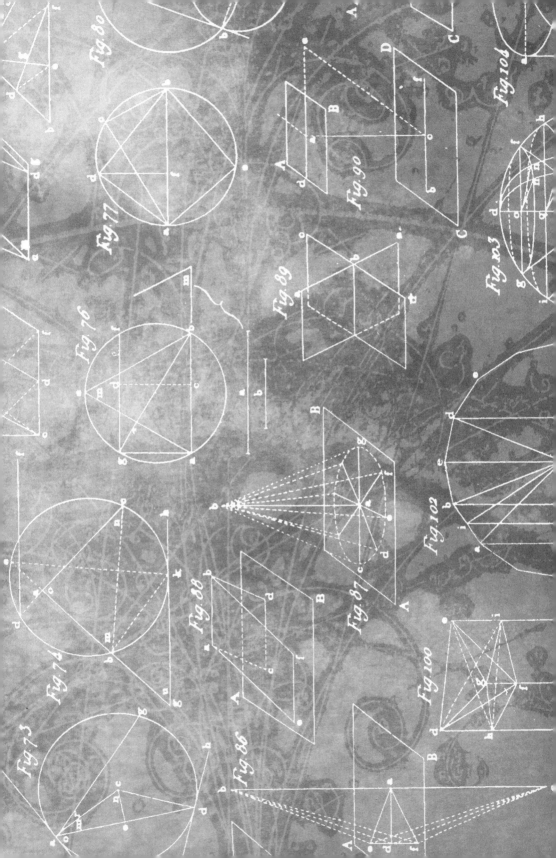

1. Origin of Life

Pan-vitalism: anima *and the cosmos*

BOURGEAULT • The origin and evolution of all life and the advent of humankind—what is sometimes called the humanization of life—have been the objects of inquiry, discussion, and debate through the centuries, and especially during the past decades.

IKEDA • These are indeed important and complex issues. The debate on some of them still continues. Since ancient times, human beings have been fascinated by the mystery of the origin of life. The result of their quest for understanding has given us no definitive answers, but rather an assortment of religious and philosophical hypotheses.

BOURGEAULT • From a philosophical viewpoint, the question of the origin of life is tied to the question of its nature. What essentially is life? What differentiates the living from the nonliving? Depending on whether they posit a radical rupture between the living and the nonliving, theories of the origin of life often belong to either a creationist or a pan-vitalist perspective.

IKEDA • When you say creationist, I suppose you are referring to theories that say life is the creation of a unique, absolute God.

BOURGEAULT • Yes, the biblical accounts relate direct, creative intervention: the origin of life depended on a divine decision—even the caprice—of a god who might just as well have refrained from creating living beings.

IKEDA • Precisely. Whether to create or not create living things depended on God's will.

BOURGEAULT • In this tradition, a divine decision explains the hierarchy observable in living things: vegetable, animal, and human. From the outset, a principle of internal cohesion—a soul—confers life on the living and determines its level—or its nature and quality.

IKEDA • And what is meant by pan-vitalism?

BOURGEAULT • Pan-vitalism holds that all parts of the universe contain the seeds of life capable of developing. In the same framework, animism refers to the concept that there are vital or spiritual forces throughout nature and the universe, imperceptible extra- or supra-natural forces that escape our attempts to observe them and remain outside our sensual perception.

IKEDA • Buddhism does not teach creation by one, absolute God. Instead, it sees the universe itself as one life entity. In this sense, it may be more akin to pan-vitalism.

We will discuss the philosophical considerations of life later. For now, I should like to examine scientific hypotheses about the origin of life. Roughly, they fall into two categories: theories that posit an extraterrestrial origin and those that posit a terrestrial origin of life.

The extraterrestrial argument

IKEDA • In 1908, Svante A. Arrhenius (1859–1927), the Swedish Nobel laureate in chemistry, made public his "panspermia" theory, according to which spores or "germs" originating on planets in the Milky Way drifted into space and "seeded" life on earth. The Russian biochemist Aleksander Oparin (1894–1980) sharply criticized the theory. Nonetheless, it aroused considerable interest in the scientific world because, since the middle of the nineteenth century, when Louis Pasteur rejected the idea of the spontaneous emergence of life, no convincing theory of the origin of life had emerged.

BOURGEAULT • But prevailing scientific thought today does not support the panspermia thesis.

IKEDA • No, there are serious objections to it. First these spores could neither have escaped the gravity of another planet nor survived the destructive radioactive bombardment and super-low temperatures of the outer-space environment. In spite of these criticisms, however, other scientists elaborated and developed the panspermia theory. One of these, the British biophysicist Francis Crick, received the Nobel Prize for Biology and Medicine, along with James Watson, for their work on DNA. Starting from the idea that all living beings on Earth share a single genetic origin, Crick posits an extraterrestrial source and the dissemination of viable spores in outer space. In the same general line of thought is the theory of British astronomer Sir Fred Hoyle (1915–) and Sri-Lankan astronomer N.C. Wickramasinghe (1939–), which seeks to establish the origins of life in comets because analysis of light from comet tails clearly reveals the presence of amino acids.

Professor Wickramasinghe, with whom I published a dialogue entitled *Space and Eternal Life*,[1] believes that the origin of DNA can be found in outer space.

BOURGEAULT · Still another theory seems at once simpler and better supported. Thanks to work of scientists, we now understand the circumstances that made possible the formation of Earth and— owing to a complex interplay of "chance and necessity," as Jacques Monod (1910–76) would say—the appearance of life there. An earthly origin of life on Earth seems more likely than an extraterrestrial one. This does not, of course, exclude the possibility that life has also emerged elsewhere under propitious conditions and owing to an interplay of chance and necessity, the definite rules of which still escape us.

IKEDA · Modern molecular biology has clearly shown that life is composed of matter like DNA and proteins. If this is the case, there is no clear demarcation between living and nonliving things. This in turn may eliminate the need to look beyond Earth for the origins of life. Even if its source is sought in outer space, we still confront the question of *how* life emerged. A continuity between living and nonliving entities allows the possibility that life began on earth.

1. *Space and Eternal Life: A Dialogue between Chandra Wickramasinghe and Daisaku Ikeda.* London: Journeyman Press. 1998.

BOURGEAULT • That seems to be the dominant trend in scientific thinking. But the Canadian astrophysicist Hubert Reeves (1932–) presents matters in a slightly different way. Instead of either a radical break between the living and the nonliving or an unbroken continuity between them, he cites a dynamic made up of both ruptures and continuity, an evolutionary dynamic that brings about an increasing complexity of entities and eventually gives rise to life. Life itself grows increasingly complex because its appearance did not impede the operation of an evolution that proceeds according to its own dynamic of ruptures and continuity. Like all other life forms and in spite of all the ruptures, human beings are made of the same material as stones and stars.

IKEDA • Reeves's apparently simple interpretation is actually very profound. It resembles the Buddhist idea that the whole universe is imbued with life and that life tendencies are observable in the birth of the Earth.

Buddhism divides all things into sentient and insentient beings. Sentient beings are living beings endowed with feelings, emotions, and consciousness. Though human beings are its most prominent members, the sentient category includes all other animals as well. Nonliving things and plants are generally categorized among insentient beings, although opinions about the inclusion of plants vary. Be that as it may, the sentient and the insentient form a continuity with human beings at one pole and minerals at the other.

The Earth, too, is regarded as a sort of living entity. The primitive, prebiological Earth, a nonliving being, is believed to have had an innate predisposition to life. The emergence of sentient beings from the insentient being of the primitive Earth and the birth of humanity are considered two parts of a continual process of evolution.

BOURGEAULT • Several years ago, I had the opportunity to attend a dialogue-conference at the University of Montreal between two famous scientists, the geneticist Albert Jacquard (1925–) and the astrophysicist Hubert Reeves.[2] The meeting of genetics and astrophysics, through these two individuals and others as well, still seems richly significant and meaningful to me today. The more we expand and deepen our understanding of ourselves and our environment—even to the cosmic level—the more we are compelled to realize that we are all parts of the same thing.

IKEDA • Yes, a common belonging based on a common origin . . . I detect a subtle scientific intuition in their theory.

Simplicity to complexity:
The process of molecular evolution

IKEDA • The commonly accepted theory of evolution arose from the idea of molecular evolution posited by the Soviet biochemist Aleksander Oparin. In 1924, at Moscow University, Oparin presented his hypothesis that life emerged on Earth as a consequence of molecular evolution. Molecular evolution means organic molecules like those of amino acids can be produced from simple inorganic molecules like those of carbon dioxide and water. Oparin scientifically demonstrated the progression from primitive organic molecules to colloidal substances to coacervated protoplasm and monocellular life forms. Later scientific research substantiated his theory.

BOURGEAULT • The American chemists Stanley Lloyd Miller (1930–) and Harold Clayton Urey (1893–1981) tried to reproduce the conditions set out in the most scientifically accepted hypotheses about the origin of life, at least on Earth. According to these theories, winds and storms would have violently disturbed the primitive oceanic soup.

IKEDA • Urey received a Nobel Prize in chemistry (1934). Miller was a graduate student at the University of Chicago, and I believe the experiment was his idea. Their joint work demonstrated the originality and flexibility of a young man and the broadmindedness and extraordinary leadership of the professor who set his young collaborator on the right path.

BOURGEAULT • In 1954, success crowned their experiment. Other scientists

2. For the text of this dialogue-conference, see "Le temps du monde fini commence: Dialogue entre Albert Jacquard et Hubert Reeves" (The era of the finite world begins: Dialogue between Albert Jacquard and Hubert Reeves) in *L'avenir d'un monde fini: jalons pour une éthique du développement durable* (The future of a finite world: Paving the way for an ethics of sustainable development). Presented by Guy Bourgeault. *Cahiers de recherche éthique*, No. 15. Montreal: Fides. 2001. 123–140.

repeated it with similar results. Submitting a mixture of liquid water and the simple gases assumed to have been present in the initial atmosphere to vigorous electrical discharges produced alcohol, sugars, fats, and amino acids.

IKEDA • Then in 1960, Professor Cyril Ponanperma (1923–) of the University of Maryland synthesized a nucleic acid base.

BOURGEAULT • Until then, such substances had been considered organic, that is, uniquely produced by living beings. This is put forth as the way the first molecules emerged on Earth, engaging in an astonishing ballet of combinations and dissociations—eventually called molecular activity—and giving rise to life forms that, by leaps and bounds, grew more complex in a ceaseless alternation of chance and necessity.

IKEDA • When Jacques Monod's book *Chance and Necessity* was published in Japanese translation in the early seventies, it caused a sensation. It was very unusual for so weighty a work to appeal to the general public. I remember reading it voraciously and pondering its message in relation to Buddhism.

BOURGEAULT • Progress has been made since its publication. Today we know more about what I call the rules of the game—what we traditionally called the laws of nature. Still, as researchers admit—indeed more willingly than the general public—many things still elude scientific analysis.

Chaos theory and the Buddhist principle of dependent causation

BOURGEAULT • What we know today about living beings and the life of living beings does not fit into the mechanist vision of, say, a Descartes (1596–1650). The living being itself is in a sense an unstable system. Does it elude science for that reason?

IKEDA • Recent molecular biology argues that all living things on Earth are carbon-based and have DNA as genetic material. Does this imply that there is some degree of inevitability involved?

BOURGEAULT • Perhaps. At least it is easier to tell ourselves that. But for twenty years American and European—especially French—scientists have been studying what has been dubbed *chaos* and thereby eliminated from all scientific consideration. James Gleick, a scientific journalist for *The New York Times,* has related the fascinating adventure of this research in a work called *Chaos*, published in 1987. It quickly became a bestseller and, since 1997, has been translated into seventeen languages. As Gleick says at the end of his book, work done during the seventies and eighties on "chaotic realities" has led to reexaminations of traditionally fundamental concepts.

IKEDA • That is an intriguing conclusion. Please tell us more about it.

BOURGEAULT • Let us take, for example, the widely accepted "fact" that simple systems behave simply, are subject to simple laws, and behave in stable, constant and therefore predictable ways, and that complex systems, on the other hand, are unstable and unpredictable. They are designated risky—here again we see chance succeeding necessity. Now analyses have shown that simple systems give rise to complex behavior and, moreover, that strange similarities—almost family ties—exist between the behaviors of different systems. The laws of complexity would thus seem universal.

IKEDA • That makes good sense.

The Chinese classic *Zhuang-zi* (fourth century BCE) contains a story relating how Chaos had once been kind to a certain man. In gratitude, the man added a nose and eyes to Chaos's hitherto featureless face. Thereupon Chaos died. The story warns that if we manipulate nature thoughtlessly, we can kill it. Nature is highly complex and delicate. If we attempt to wrestle it into the box of necessity, we may destroy it in the long term.

Buddhism sees all existence in terms of the principle of dependent causation. Everything emerges and recedes as a result of mutual relations between direct and contributory causes. Some of the most important causal relationships are considered to be examples of necessity or inevitability, but Buddhist thought takes account of the interplay between chance and inevitability in the relationships between beings and phenomena and other beings and phenomena. In consequence, and given the Buddhist perspective of dependent causation, we are not bound by a dichotomy between the inevitable and the accidental. The important thing is to remember that, as you say, both simple and complex entities behave in complex ways.

BOURGEAULT • Here we see something truly revolutionary or—to return to words spoken by Thomas Kuhn when he was studying *The Structure of Scientific Revolutions*—a paradigm shift.[3] It is not by chance but by necessity and in order to fully account for their work that scientists in various fields have been led, in the past two decades, to abolish the boundaries between disciplines and increase interdisciplinary and transdisciplinary interaction.

IKEDA • The dialogue between geneticist Albert Jacquard and astrophysicist Hubert Reeves that you mentioned earlier is a good example.

BOURGEAULT • Precisely. We could cite many other names and many other encounters. Once perceived, the complexity of reality requires boundaries between disciplines to be broken down. It is impossible to truly comprehend anything in reality without taking into account the dynamic play of interactions and the strikingly complex networks of interdependent factors that appear to proliferate upon each closer examination. New, "universal" rules and laws—that is, functioning and observable in various fields and at various levels of complexity—seem to rule the game.

In the 1960s, Joël de Rosnay examined the question of the origins of life. He gradually came to realize that advances in knowledge about those origins are due largely to discoveries made possible by two important instruments: the telescope and the microscope.[4] To make further observations, suggested de Rosnay, who was working with both the Pasteur Institute in Paris and the Massachusetts Institute of Technology in Boston, humankind needs a third instrument, which he called the macroscope (after his widely read book).[5] The macroscope would enable us to thoroughly understand the interactions and interdependencies of the complex systemic networks that link all beings to each other.

3. Thomas Kuhn. *The Structure of Scientific Revolutions.* Chicago: University of Chicago Press. 1962.
4. Joël de Rosnay. *Origines de la vie.* Paris: Éditions du Seuil. 1966.
5. Joël de Rosnay. *The Macroscope.* Tr. Robert Edwards. New York: Harper & Row. 1977.

In a more recent book entitled *Symbiotic Man: A New Understanding of the Organization of Life and a Vision of the Future,*[6] de Rosnay argues that tomorrow's humankind will exist in close symbiosis with a planetary organism we are now constructing through complex communications networks that constitute the nervous system of the new planetary entity.

IKEDA • The macroscope is an intriguing idea for a scientific elucidation of the interdependence of all existence.

2. Theories of Biological Evolution

Darwin and natural selection

IKEDA • More than 140 years have gone by since Charles Darwin (1809–82) published *The Origin of the Species by Means of Natural Selection, or The Preservation of Favored Races in the Struggle for Life.* Since then, the theory of biological evolution and natural selection that it propounds has had an immense impact not only on biology, but on all of society.

BOURGEAULT • And yet the Darwinian theory seems simplistic to us today.

IKEDA • Yes it does. Darwin's theory was hailed in the history of biological evolution as the first to postulate an evolutionary mechanism. Today, however, it is being re-evaluated from various angles in the light of recent advances in molecular biology and molecular genetics.

BOURGEAULT • The true value of his theory is that it occasioned, in its own time, research and vigorous discussion, less in defense of evolutionary theory against the established tenets of creationism than in search of a better understanding of the modalities of evolution, which was already backed by significant evidence.

---

6. Joël de Rosnay. *Symbiotic Man: A New Understanding of the Organization of Life and a Vision of the Future.* Tr. Phyllis Aronoff. New York: MacGraw-Hill. 2000.

IKEDA • Before we delve more deeply into the theory, I would like to state the main elements of Darwinian evolution that our discussion will be based on. First, living things generally reproduce in large numbers. Second, these large numbers give rise to fierce competition for survival. Third, mutations occurring in some offspring sometimes prove advantageous in the competition for survival. Fourth, the mutated subjects have an increased possibility of surviving, however slight. And fifth, after centuries and millennia of repetitions of this process, the mutated forms come to account for the majority of the species, thus producing a new species.

BOURGEAULT • Yes, but some of Darwin's assertions are far from being as simple as that.

IKEDA • True. If we simplify his idea schematically as "prolific reproduction—struggle for survival—natural selection—evolution," as you say, some aspects of the mechanism remain unclear. He offers no scientific explanation of the actual form the struggle for survival takes, the frequency with which mutations occur, or the precise genetic mechanism.

BOURGEAULT • Actually, Darwinism and neo-Darwinism have turned out to be more interesting in many respects than Darwin's own proposals.

IKEDA • Knowledge of genetics increased rapidly in the twentieth century, leading to the emergence of neo-Darwinism, or general evolutionary theory. It is difficult to say exactly who first set out the theory, but based on work on mutations by the Dutch botanist Hugo De Vries (1848–1935) and on genetics by the Austrian botanist Gregor Mendel (1822–84), scientists began to answer several questions that Darwin's original theory left unanswered. Since general evolutionary theory goes beyond Darwin's framework, which claims evolution is fundamentally the result of natural selection, it is called neo-Darwinism.

BOURGEAULT • I could easily make a list of improper uses made of Darwin's ideas on the survival of the fittest through natural selection. They have been wrongly transferred to socio-politics to legitimize Nazi practices and, more recently, dyed-in-the-wool partisan neoliberalism that supports free enterprise leading to the triumph of the most powerful. But these misuses have not been entirely surprising.

To a great extent, the fate of Darwin's theory and Darwinism is the result of their having been developed in the context of a booming industrial society and a liberal ideology championing rivalry and competition. Today we understand the influence context exerts on scientific works of all kinds and on the way we view problems. We can interpret the application of Darwinism to social and political planes as a boomerang effect.

IKEDA • It is damaging to science to apply natural scientific hypotheses directly to human society. Interpreting ideas like natural selection and the survival of the fittest as permission to victimize the weak is unpardonable.

Human beings are prone to think that misfortune happens only to others. But as the American psychologist Carl R. Rogers (1901–87) pointed out, danger pursues all living creatures. Nonetheless, people go on thinking that incidents that leave a deep scar in the soul will never happen to them. This is what the psychologist Linda S. Perloff calls the "illusion of immortality."

The young prince Shakyamuni, striving to break with illusions, objectively studied himself, others, and the environment, and forced himself to overcome the sufferings of existence in the most radical way. Even before rejecting the secular world at the age of nineteen, Shakyamuni was conscious that he must never be haughty and arrogant toward the weak, even though he was in a position of strength, because he realized that at any time he could become one of the weak. The famous story of the "four encounters" symbolizes the fact that human beings cannot escape from the four sorrows of birth, aging, illness, and death. After coming to this realization, Shakyamuni set out on a spiritual quest, making compassion the basic principle he lived by and insisting on the right of the weak to live with dignity.

BOURGEAULT • It is impossible to set too high a value on compassion for the weak.

IKEDA • In reality, however, aggressive individuals and groups are ready to blindly and impulsively attack the weak, basing their actions on the theories of survival of the fittest and natural selection. The weak are pushed to the margins of society for as long as they remain weak. They must strengthen themselves and become wise. It is through experience and effort that people grow; acquired skills are much more important than natural skills.

I believe in the need for education in all sectors of society, to help the weak strengthen their defenses against the strong.

Internal dynamic, interactive dynamic

BOURGEAULT • To return to Darwin, scientific opinion of the importance of his works and his writings on the evolution of living beings is divided. As André Pichot observed in his book *L'histoire de la notion de vie* (History of the idea of life),[7] Darwin's success arises not from his explanation of evolution, but from his *not* explaining evolution and contenting himself with taking it into consideration in a fairly loose way. Thanks to this lack of constraint, molecular biology was able to develop freely.

You are quite right to say that, by confirming and correcting and adding to Darwin's theories and, more generally, Darwinism and neo-Darwinism, later breakthroughs in molecular and population genetics have surpassed them both and assured their place in scientific thought.

IKEDA • If I understand correctly, other theories have arisen in opposition to Darwinian evolution. For instance, neutral evolution holds that the majority of sudden mutations are neither advantageous nor disadvantageous to living creatures but are only neutral changes. The punctuated-equilibrium theory holds that evolution is not a continuing process but arises as a result of sudden changes over short periods, which are followed by long periods free of change. Although these new theories present hypotheses distinctly different from Darwinism, they, too, remain incomplete and require further proof.

Let us take a closer look at questions at the center of the debate on biological evolution. (1) Are the acquired traits transmitted hereditarily? (2) Does environment or heredity play the major role in evolution? (3) Is evolution an orchestrated, inevitable outcome or a matter of pure chance? (4) Is evolution continuous or intermittent? (5) Which

---

7. André Pichot. *L'histoire de la notion de vie*. Paris: Éditions Gallimard. 1993.

is more important, conciliation with circumstances as they are or competing with circumstances in order to survive?

BOURGEAULT · The questions you have succinctly formulated are in a sense obligatory, or at least constantly posed, in discussions of the evolution of living things. But they cannot be given definitive answers unless we are able to reply with a categorical yes to one alternative and an equally categorical no to the other—transmissible versus non-transmissible characteristics, teleology versus material and mechanistic determinism, chance versus necessity, competition versus adaptation, and so on. I think that giving such categorical answers is either not possible—at least no longer possible—or largely unfruitful and only faintly heuristic.

As I have already tried to explain, unless we take into account the complexity of beings, especially living beings, their organization and their situations, it is impossible to understand them—impossible to understand their "nature," as the ancient philosophers would say—or, by extension, their internal dynamics and interactive dynamic with others.

IKEDA · I see your point. We must turn our attention to what you call the internal, interactive dynamism of living beings at the base of evolution. With that in mind, I should like to go over some hotly debated issues.

The French naturalist Lamarck (1744–1829) argued that traits acquired as a result of the external environment could be hereditarily transmitted and that this was an element in evolution. Many scientists reject this theory, but the American Nobel laureate (1975) in medicine and physiologist Howard M. Temin (1934–) has advanced the idea that, though there is still no proof, retroviruses may manifest a mechanism for hereditary transmission of acquired traits.[8]

BOURGEAULT · We have long believed that only what was hereditarily received could be hereditarily transmitted; that is, only the innate—not the acquired—could be passed on from generation to generation.

---

8. Retroviruses possess an enzyme for converting RNA into DNA. They can insert their own genes into those of other animals, including human beings, and this may be the mechanism for hereditarily transmitting acquired traits.

Perhaps this idea, too, was self-generated at a time when land inherited from the father was preserved undivided to be later transmitted to the grandson.

In biology and genetics, we must bear in mind changes from one generation to another—mutations—and try to explain them. For instance, we must try to explain why young North Americans today are taller than their parents. In this case, exchanges between living beings and their environment prove decisive. Changes in food and life style explain, in part, the observed transformation. In reality, however, the situation is decidedly more complex than the established rules—which must constantly be re-examined—allow us to foresee.

Inevitable or accidental?

IKEDA · Whether environment or the living being—in other words, heredity—plays the lead role is another question scientists tussle with in a conflict between what you call teleology and mechanistic determinism. Does the evolution of living beings serve the purposes of life or is it the mechanical reaction to changes in the environment? What is your opinion?

BOURGEAULT · Teleology or mechanistic determinism? The notion of a program—or perhaps the image or allegory of a program that I will outline in a moment—prompts us to re-examine the relationship, in the advent and evolution of life, between what is given—which is both predetermined and determinant—and what is to be accomplished, constructed or brought to maturity. Implicitly, both teleology and mechanistic determinism reflect a program that, in turn, reflects an intention. In the deterministic view, nothing can appear that was not already somehow present—written in advance, inscribed in the living being, ineluctable. In a sense, the internal "program" is closed.

IKEDA · In terms of a philosophical concept, this sounds like fatalism. The fate of the living being is determined from the outset, and there is no margin of freedom.

BOURGEAULT · In the teleological view, the program is outside the living being. It exerts a sort of "remote control" over development and evolution. This program is open, not closed, since the design, even though not apparent—and here we return even more neatly to the idea of intention—inexorably, if discreetly, sets out the route to be followed.

IKEDA · The teleological view has something in common with the idea of control of destiny by God, the Creator, on the basis of whose plan changes in the universe take place. Some Japanese Buddhist sects and new religions assert the importance of realizing that an absolute being—a god or Buddha—grants and maintains human life. Their point of view leaves no room for the autonomy of human existence, that is, for the notion that we follow our own direction.

To be sure, no human can live entirely independently. We depend on nature and society for our basic needs. In this sense, our lives are granted and maintained by something other than ourselves, and we should be grateful to that "something" that makes life possible. Apart from this, to add significance to our lives we must generate value that we ourselves create, and for that we must preserve our autonomy and contribute to our social and natural environment by the creation of nobler values. The teleological approach deprives the individual living entity of freedom and closes the door on independent creative activity.

BOURGEAULT · No doubt you are right. In the teleological view, no matter how things seem, everything is controlled by necessity. Nothing is left to chance. Really, however, the role of chance seems to have been decisive in the evolutionary dynamic.

IKEDA · It is chance that gives us freedom and the possibility of creativity. Which leads us to the question of whether evolution is accidental or inevitable.

BOURGEAULT · In this connection, I shall draw freely on a message presented at a May 1994 conference on "Medicine and Philosophy" by Henri Atlan (1931–), a biophysicist at the Hôtel-Dieu de Paris. Professor Atlan showed how, in our quest to understand and develop the theory of genetics, the computer can serve as a useful metaphor to help articulate the observable stable and changing elements in all living beings. The metaphor works from two angles, depending on whether emphasis is placed on the program or the data. On the one hand there is the fixed, the predetermined, that is, the program. On the other there are the changing, unforeseen, even unforeseeable data. In short, order and disorder. Here, in apparently inverse relation, we encounter the interplay of the dynamic interactions—characteristic of living beings—of the chance and necessity that Jacques Monod spoke of. We see clearly how insufficient the image or allegory of the program is. And this revives secular philosophical debates about the relationship between being and movement, essence and existence, and nature and nurture.

Competition or conciliation?

IKEDA • As a Buddhist, I accept the thesis that, under the influence of both necessity and chance, evolution alters and develops within a continuous, dynamic mutual operation. The issue of competition or conciliation, the last of our questions, probably cannot be dealt with in an either-or fashion, either. Even so, I would like to bring up the Japanese anthropologist Kinji Imanishi, who has proposed an original theory of evolution opposed to Darwinian competition for survival. Imanishi argues that among living beings of the same species, competition is weak because there are no essential differences, and so adaptation—or what he calls "biotope segregation" based on habitat—takes precedence.

When Imanishi's article appeared in *Nature* in 1986, he caught the attention of experts the world over. His theory is based on habitat segregation and the "species society," concepts drawn from his observations of a species of mayfly living around the Kamogawa River in Kyoto. Imanishi holds that the species, not the individual, is the basic evolutionary unit and, rejecting natural selection and the idea of competition and survival of the fittest, he emphasizes the role of habitat and puts forth adaptation and biotope segregation as the basic evolutionary process. Imanishi's detractors say that his theory fails to specify the mechanism of evolutionary change.

BOURGEAULT • On one hand, we have competition and war, and on the other, adjustment or adaptation to ecological niches. In my view, these two opposed dynamics have always been at work in human history, by turns and sometimes simultaneously.

IKEDA • Certainly competition and conciliation have appeared in a wide variety of forms in human history.

BOURGEAULT • We have made war to enlarge our territory, annexing land from which we have driven indigenous inhabitants. We have conquered so-called new worlds and exploited their resources without concerning ourselves with either the wishes or the imminent fate of the local residents. But I shouldn't be speaking in the past tense. Part of our current dynamic is the tribal struggles and destructive civil wars currently tearing so many countries apart, and competition among big transnational companies that becomes outright commercial warfare, eliminating the weakest.

IKEDA • Very clearly put. It is true that both competition and conciliation have helped weave the fabric of human history. Now, however, as we face innumerable and intertwined global issues, we must radically change gear and turn away from war and toward cooperation and harmonious coexistence.

Autonomy of living organisms

BOURGEAULT • Earlier I deliberately emphasized the continuity between matter and life. Recent developments in biology—especially in molecular biology and genetics—have clearly demonstrated how living beings are subject to the same physico-chemical laws as nonliving things. But, as André Pichot has said, overemphasizing continuity runs the risk of depriving biology of its subject matter: diversity of life and living beings. We must therefore take into consideration the ruptures as well.

The living being is subject to the same physico-chemical laws as nonliving things. Living beings "live" those laws, integrate them and manage them in their own ways. We must recognize the evolutionary non-continuity—at least in certain regards—between the living and the nonliving, and perhaps also between different classes of living things, in order to make room in a consistent theory for the autonomy of the living being and its necessary exchanges with its milieu.

For exchanges to take place, there must be a community of belonging, a shared submission to physico-chemical laws. At the same time, discontinuity is necessary for the specific integration of exterior contributions into a new dynamic of autonomous evolution. Without such a rupture, the living being ceases to be: only a cadaver remains.

IKEDA • Buddhism recognizes both continuity and discontinuity between the sentient and insentient, and teaches that sentient beings can emerge from insentient beings. It explains the continuity and discontinuity between the sentient and the insentient in this way. Both the sentient and the insentient are made up of the temporary combination of what are called the five components of life—form, perception, conception, volition, and consciousness. The five components temporarily unite to constitute individual beings, both sentient and insentient.

If form (material existence) is manifest and the other four components remain latent, the combination results in insentience. In biological evolution, through continuous interaction with the environment, the four other latent components gradually became manifest.

Perception is the function that receives information through the six sense organs (the five senses plus the coordinating "intellect"). Conception is the function that creates ideas or mental images based on what was perceived. Finally, volition is the will that acts on the mental images and motivates an action in response to what was perceived.

In addition to form, animals are endowed with perception, conception and will. Plants, too, are now thought to have perception, that is, sensitivity and emotion. It was only with the advent of humanity that the fifth component—consciousness—emerged. The autonomy or identity of humankind is firmly rooted in this function of discernment. In sum, I am in basic agreement with what you say about the autonomy of living beings and exchanges between them and their environments.

3. Birth of Humankind

Genetic analysis sheds lights on human evolution

IKEDA • Here we are at last at the birth of humanity, following a complex discussion of the evolution of life. But the appearance of humankind is an equally complex topic. Darwin's assertion that "man descended from apes" stirred up quite a controversy at the time.

BOURGEAULT · Yes, but it is hard to say when and how the growing complexity of life introduced such breaks in the dynamic evolutionary continuity.

IKEDA · Until recently, fossils provided the sole scientific proof of human origins. But now rapid advances in molecular biology allow scientists to date the phases of evolution through genetic analysis.

Genes store mutations accumulated over hundreds of millions of years of evolution. By comparing the amino acid sequences of different species (which are genetically determined by DNA), we can calculate how long they have been separated from a common ancestor.

Using protein sequences and DNA, it has been possible to devise a sort of molecular clock to measure evolution. It can show us how a specific evolutionary ramification occurred (what split off from what) and when the split occurred. The more differences found in the amino acid sequence, the more distantly related the species in question.

BOURGEAULT · For a moment, let us go much farther back in time, using results of the most recent research. The Big Bang is estimated to have taken place about 15 billion years ago—or even more if we accept newer studies. Life "emerged" from matter about three billion years ago. Hominids made their appearance recently: only 3.5 million years ago or perhaps a little more according to a recent discovery in Africa. With *Australopithecus afarensis* (notably the fossil remains dubbed Lucy), our ancestors became bipedal. This stage was apparently important to the advent of the human being as known to us today.

IKEDA · V.M. Sarich and A.C. Wilson of the University of California used molecular clocks to study primate evolution and came to the conclusion that humanoids branched from the gorillas and chimpanzees eight or nine million years ago. Given the time required for evolution to take them to the hominid bipedal stage, I think your estimation of the time scale is correct.

BOURGEAULT · Still closer to us, about two million years ago, appeared Java man and Peking man (both representatives of *Homo erectus*) and then *Homo habilis*. As the paleontologist Yvon Pageau notes,[9] to

9. Yvon Pageau. *Le phénomène humain et l'évolution* (The human phenomenon and evolution). Montreal: Éditions du Méridien. 1990.

stretch out his hand and speak, man first had to take a step. The first humans were set apart by their manual skills in fashioning stone tools and by the growth of their cranial volume and complexity. Next came the ability to speak and the discovery of fire. The adventure that is human history starts with these events.

IKEDA • There are two basic theories about the origins of humankind: one holds that the evolutionary descent from primates occurred in many different places around the world, and the other claims that it occurred in one place only. I gather you agree with the second hypothesis, the African origin of our species. Certain factors do support the one-place theory. For example, fossils of *Homo sapiens* have been discovered only in Africa. In addition, molecular-genetic data have revealed little difference in the genes of Caucasoids, Mongoloids, and Negroids.

Imparting meaning to life and human consciousness

IKEDA • We have broached the advent of the human species from a biological viewpoint, but when it comes to the emergence of humanity—not merely as *Homo sapiens* but in the fullest humane sense— the ideas of biological evolution are insufficient. Of course, we are animals; but we are more than simple living organisms. We can create cultures and build societies. We are reflective, introspective creatures capable of self-control through autonomous thought and reason and spirituality.

BOURGEAULT • The preparatory stages took a long time. But you are right: with the human being, something new took shape.

IKEDA • I would like to bring up a topic that has fascinated me for some time now. Remains excavated by Dr. Ralph Solecki at Shanidar in Iraq suggest that the Neanderthals conducted burials and sprinkled corpses with flowers. If this is true, they had already advanced beyond the animal stage and could view death introspectively and reflectively. Incidentally, scholarly opinion holds that the Neanderthals became extinct and have no relation to modern human beings.

BOURGEAULT • This is an important point. The novelty manifested or revealed in Neanderthal rituals is the ability to give meaning to life. The same capacity is demonstrated by the Cro-Magnon drawings dating back ten or twelve thousand years in the caverns of Altamira in Spain and Lascaux in France and others, dating back perhaps twenty-five or even thirty thousand years in the Chauvet cave at Ardeche in France. Giving meaning to one's own life, to the lives of other humans and of other living beings, and ultimately to the cosmic adventure itself, which we have been recounting—this is the foundation for culture.

IKEDA • In *The Sickness Unto Death*, Kierkegaard (1813–55) states that man is spirit, that spirit is self, and that self is the relationship each individual has with himself—that is, self-consciousness. Buddhism makes a detailed analysis of the structure of self-consciousness. The Consciousness-Only school posits four divisions of consciousness: the object of consciousness, direct consciousness of that object, the self that is aware of this direct consciousness, and the self that is aware of that conscious self. This last self-conscious self can be said to engage in internal dialogue with the self.

Walking upright, using tools and fire, expressing ourselves artistically and verbally, these are indeed characteristics of humankind. But self-consciousness, a trait inherent in human life, makes these characteristics possible. Henri Bergson (1859–1941) said that, in the narrow sense, tools are products of the intellect. In other words, self-consciousness as a spiritual structure is unique to human beings. It is the very foundation of human nature as distinct from animal nature.

BOURGEAULT • Without doubt, the capacity to give life meaning depends on consciousness, that is, the ability to be aware of ourselves and to know we are alive. It brings to mind the image of a mirror, reflecting and showing us ourselves as we live and then permitting us to choose, within certain constraints, the orientation we desire.

Just as there is a rupture, despite the continuity, between the nonliving and the living, so, no doubt, is there another between the living non-human (the animal) and the human. Certainly we can find many non-human species with the capacity to react and adapt to their environments. The complex social organizations and behaviors we observe in ants, birds, whales, and porpoises bear witness to this. These observations add weight to theories that emphasize continuity and blood ties.

Continuity and rupture

IKEDA • In Buddhist terms, non-human animals can be assumed to possess the perception, conception, and volition I talked about earlier. They even manifest the consciousness that integrates these three with the fourth component of life, form—at least in part. In the light of this similarity, it is possible to recognize continuity between human and non-human animals.

BOURGEAULT • Continuity, yes, but how do you explain the ruptures?

IKEDA • Very conceivably, though *conditioned* by material mechanisms, biological life activities are not *determined* by them. The Australian physiologist Sir John Carew Eccles (1903–1997) suggested that even the creative process of evolution is incapable of bridging the gap between the physico-chemical processes of the cerebral cortex and the psychological processes of consciousness.

Similarly, the Canadian brain specialist Dr. W. G. Penfield (1891–1976) wrote that somehow or other, nerve stimulation is transformed into thought and thought becomes nerve stimulation. This much we know for sure. But the knowledge does nothing to explain the essential nature of our wonderful minds.

BOURGEAULT • Referring to language and thought, some people locate the specifically human element in the soul or spirit. Others see no need to resort to the spirit to account for something related to novel possibilities in a more complex living organization. Penfield was not the first to make such an assessment; that is, to measure the physico-chemistry of human thought, sentiment, and emotion. But thought—or consciousness, to get back to our exact topic—is possible only because of the functioning of the complex organism that is the human being—more specifically because of the functioning of the human brain.

Now, we can study and measure brain function or activity according to ordinary physical and chemical rules. For instance, today we use lithium to treat manic-depression by reducing and controlling excessive deviations of enthusiasm and anxiety. And this brings us back to the manifest continuity—in spite of the ruptures—of matter and life, of matter and consciousness.

IKEDA • I have already mentioned the Buddhist concept of the oneness of body and mind (*shikishin-funi*). The Japanese term for inseparability or oneness derives from the expression that means "two but not two (*nini-funi*)." "Two" indicates the separate functions of the body and the mind, denoting discontinuity or rupture. "Not two (*funi*)," on the other hand, indicates unity and indivisibility, denoting the continuity of matter and spirit.

In the treatment of manic-depression you just mentioned, the mind is a unified *psychological* system. Lithium physically and chemically influences the brain, the nervous system and the other bodily organs which comprise a unified *physiological* system. Physical and chemical changes in the body influence mental state. By like token, anxiety and worry influence hormone secretion, thus affecting physical and chemical conditions such as body temperature. The psychological and physical systems are distinct yet they influence each other, and the Buddhist concept of "two but not two" considers them indivisibly one. A similar relationship exists between the individual and the environment.

Consciousness of the self and of the eternal

BOURGEAULT • What do we mean by *matter* and *spirit*? Should we not realize that what we call spirit is only perceptible, in fact, only exists through matter, which is not, as is sometimes said, merely the substratum or support of the spirit but its "seat" and its necessary and unique location? It seems to me that we underestimate matter in both the living being—including humans—and in spiritual consciousness. Dichotomous thinking compels us to choose between realities that it would be better to reconcile and connect.

The novelty that emerged with the advent of the human being— and perhaps still more with our subsequent development—is the capacity to impart meaning to life. Meaning thus imparted is a mark not only of human life, both as individuals and as history-creating societies, but also of the future of the world itself.

IKEDA • When I think of the evolution of life in its entirety, I am inclined to think that, for self-awareness to emerge, humans had to define the position of the self in relation to the eternal universe. In other words, the mechanism of introspective, reflective self-awareness was possible only when human beings began to think about their position in relation to the universe and consider an eternal force propelling cosmic evolution. As I see it, this development constituted a creative input into cosmic biological evolution. From the standpoint of human evolution, it signified the return of humankind to the cosmos through an internal transcendence of physical evolution—an encounter with the eternal. Existential angst and fear are nothing other than the subconscious emotions arising from the encounter between the finite self and the infinite eternal. This is where religion begins.

Buddhism teaches that self-awareness arises through our encounters with the eternal. Buddhism urges us to be receptive to the most profound meaning of living, in the eternal process of cosmic evolution, and further urges that we accept, as our mission, compassionate behavior toward all beings. The consciousness that the existence of all living beings in the vast space of the universe is a function of the same creative evolutionary process of interactions that includes our own existence. This awareness is exactly what gives meaning to life and helps us transcend the abyss of life and death.

4. Diverse Views

Changing perceptions of life and social structures

IKEDA • We have explored the origins of life, the evolution of living beings and the emergence of humankind. Now I suggest we discuss the diversity of views on life. I would like to know what life means for you.

BOURGEAULT • What is life? We have certainly not conclusively answered that question. From the opening pages of his monumental *L'histoire de la notion de vie* (The history of the idea of life), Pichot asserts that, though it affects us closely, the idea of life has never been clearly defined in the histories of either science or philosophy. We are aware of ourselves and of being alive. But perhaps because life constantly renews itself and simultaneously renews our consciousness and knowledge of it, it seems to escape our definition. Pichot goes on to remark that we might say of life what Augustine, Bishop of Hippo at the beginning of the fifth century, said of time: I know what it is as long as no one asks me about it. But if I am asked to explain it, I no longer know what it is. At the outset, therefore, I confess my own ignorance of what my whole being knows from daily experience.

IKEDA • We *are* life. And yet we are hard put to define it. It reminds me of something Linus Pauling, with whom I held a dialogue,[10] once told an international academic conference: it is easier to study life than to define it. We can study it without defining it. This seems very sensible to me.

BOURGEAULT • There are diverse ways of being and living in the world. These "ways of being" vary from person to person, from group to group, from society to society, and from epoch to epoch. This is why, as you insist, there are diverse conceptions of life. Our conception of life seems profoundly related to social structures, especially to modalities of power-sharing within a society.

IKEDA • Are you suggesting that social structures influence the way we view life?

BOURGEAULT • In highly hierarchical societies and at times when interior social divisions have seemed necessary to society's survival—or at least to the maintenance of the established order—the origin and evolution of life have been presented in terms of stages and rigidly hierarchical orders. The great Biblical myth of the creation, describing order emerging progressively from chaos and establishing or justifying existing hierarchies, is a case in point. The Bible first speaks of inorganic matter, then of organic matter, living creatures, and finally humanity at the pinnacle of a pyramid, the lower levels of which are subjugated by the superior ones. God created, day by day and in this order, the light of day, which he separated from the shadows of night; the sky, from which descend the waters; the earth, which he separated from the waters under the firmament and caused to produce grasses

10. *A Lifelong Quest for Peace: A Dialogue.* Sudbury, Mass.: Jones and Bartlett Publishers, Inc. 1992.

and fruit trees; living beings that swarm in the seas and fly in the air under the lights of day and night; animals called upon to multiply on Earth; and finally man and his companion, to whom he gave the mandate to cultivate and subdue the universe. Later, in order to classify objects for observation, people distinguished three orders—mineral, vegetable, and animal. The human being belongs to but transcends the third order.

IKEDA · Then, as scientific knowledge increases and social structures alter, views of life, too, change.

BOURGEAULT · Yes. And that is why modern societies, more democratically oriented and therefore less hierarchical than their predecessors, are more given to an awareness of common belonging and solidarity than to hierarchical distinctions. This has important repercussions on our conception of life—especially human life—and the significance we impart to it.

In terms of life and its origins—or the relationship between life and matter, between the animate and the inanimate—a new sensitivity stresses continuities more than ruptures, interdependencies more than autonomies. The titles of two recent works of popular science are revealing in this connection: *Poussières d'étoiles*[11] (Stardust) by Hubert Reeves and *Vital Dust: Life as a Cosmic Imperative*[12] by Christian de Duve (1917–).

In another book entitled *Patience dans l'azur*[13] (Patience in the sky), Reeves describes the slow maturation process that has taken place in an uninterrupted development of complexity of matter since the Big Bang 15 billion years ago. In *Vital Dust*, proceeding in the opposite direction, de Duve focuses on the evolution of life by tracing the path from the complex to the simple in what precedes the human: the components of life.

These conceptions of life grant pre-eminence to continuities rather than discontinuities and to interdependence rather than autonomy.

11. Hubert Reeves. *Poussières d'étoiles*. Paris: Éditions du Seuil. 1984.
12. Christian de Duve. *Vital Dust: Life as a Cosmic Imperative*. New York: Basic Books. 1995.
13. Hubert Reeves. *Patience dans l'azur*. Paris: Éditions du Seuil. 1981.

The Cartesian view of life:
Cosmology and physics of Descartes's era

IKEDA • As you point out, views of life have shifted from hierarchies and autonomies to solidarities and interdependencies.

The currently-prevailing view of life is the mechanistic view. It is premised on the idea that life emerged from matter and remains material while displaying functions that are immaterial. The positivist study of life depends on this premise—that physical matter can display immaterial functions—in order to overturn the view that life springs from life and support the view that life sprang from matter. During the past three decades, life research has made astounding progress. New knowledge of genetics, heredity, immunity and brain function, to name just a few, have opened incredible vistas of the behavior of matter at the molecular level—remarkable behavior never before observed in ordinary physical matter.

Dr. Bourgeault, what are your thoughts on the mechanistic view of life since the time of Descartes?

BOURGEAULT • We can more easily understand the general orientations of Descartes's thought if we put it in parallel with Galilean conceptions. In demonstrating the double movement of the planets—revolving on their own axes and orbiting around the sun—Copernicus (1473–1543) opened the way for Galileo's (1564–1642) work, and especially for the construction and elaboration of his mechanical theories. Descartes's conception of life—his biology—can be clearly understood only in reference to Copernican cosmology and Galilean physics as influenced by the mechanist paradigm. Astral movement is explained and interpreted according to the model—the mechanics—of a clock. This model furnished a key to the comprehension of the physical world, its functioning, and living beings—specifically human beings, with which Descartes's biology is almost exclusively concerned.

IKEDA • Descartes recognized in human beings a characteristic not found in other living beings; that is, the ability to think. His philosophy is a dualism between "extent"—the physical space commanded by the living being—and thought. For non-human living beings, the monism of extent suffices.

BOURGEAULT • According to Descartes, the human being is composed of two distinct substances that biology can never successfully unite: extension (the body) and consciousness (the soul). Here he breaks definitively with the Aristotelian vision of the soul as a form of the body and the living being—all living beings—and as an internal principle of movement that allows the living being to develop autonomously, if I may put it that way. The idea that the animal and vegetable kingdoms had no soul, already suggested by Galen, reached its culmination with Descartes.

According to him, only human beings have souls. As Georges Canguilhem said in *La connaissance de la vie* (The knowledge of life),[14] Descartes did for animals what Aristotle (384–322 BCE) did for slaves: he depreciated them to justify their use as tools. The venture called civilization would lead the West to consider man—and to try to make him—master and proprietor of nature, including the human body and humanity itself. With the development of genetics and the demands of licensed property rights on modified genetic combinations or sequences, we may go still farther down this path.

Contemporary effect of the mechanistic vision

IKEDA • Recent dramatic advances in molecular biology suggest that we will indeed go farther. Science is now dabbling in the realm of the soul. These developments attest to the enormous success of the mechanistic view of life since Descartes's time.

We may call it a mechanistic view of life, but "mechanistic" embraces a variety of concepts. Sometimes it is used to describe a methodology of classifying living phenomena with vague reference to the classical notions of dynamics. It can also express a conviction that living phenomena can be reduced to biology or chemistry. Sometimes it indicates only an analogy with artificial machines.

All these variations are founded on the belief that there is only matter at the basis of all living phenomena and that therefore life is no more than matter behaving in a particular way. This mechanistic premise, however, is neither self-evident nor completely proven.

14. Georges Canguilhem. *La connaissance de la vie.* Paris: Vrin. 1969.

BOURGEAULT • Perhaps, but we must remember that Descartes cleared the way for modern biomedicine. In retrospect, that was his goal in constructing the Cartesian mechanical model of the living body—including humans.

According to Descartes, the human body—if not the whole human being—is a machine. His *Treatise of Man* (1662) contains the following description—now considered classic—of the animal-machine or the imaginary automaton that nonetheless resembles the real human body.

"I assume their body to be but a statue, an earthen machine formed intentionally by God to be as much as possible like us. Thus, not only does He give it externally the shapes and colors of all the parts of our bodies; He also places inside it all the pieces required to make it walk, eat, breathe, and imitate whichever of our functions can be imagined to precede from mere matter and to depend entirely on the arrangement of our organs.

"We see clocks, artificial fountains, mills, and similar machines which, though made entirely by man, lack not the power to move, of themselves, in various ways. And I think you will agree that the present machine could have even more sorts of movement than I have imagined and more ingenuity than I have assigned, for our supposition is that it was created by God."[15]

While we can say that Descartes understands the living human being—at least the human body—according to a machine model, we must remember that the machine itself is a creation of humankind and to an extent is constructed on a human model. Fundamentally then, the mechanistic vision or conception of the living being and of life itself remains anthropomorphic. As Canguilhem noted, Descartes simply replaced the political anthropomorphism in vogue at that time with technological anthropomorphism.

IKEDA • Therefore, there is no reason we should refuse to recognize the validity of non-mechanistic theories of life. As the Swiss zoologist Adolph Portman (1897–1982) said, a pluralist viewpoint is essential to the study of life forms. No one view is more important or more

15. René Descartes. *Treatise on Man.* Tr. Thomas Steele Hall. Cambridge: Harvard Monographs in the History of Science. 1972.

scientific than any other. So it is not surprising that, to counter the mechanistic vision, the very mainstay of modern science, other methods of studying life have been proposed, based for example on subjective experience.

BOURGEAULT • The view proposed by Descartes is, of course, only one construct among many, but it had its own particular destiny. Pre-Cartesian views arranged life forms—or orders or stages—hierarchically. In doing so they reflected and consolidated the social orders and power relationships in force at that time. By leveling, on a theoretical plane, the hierarchy of life forms within the dynamic of the mechanistic paradigm, the Cartesian vision prepares the way for, and in a sense legitimizes, the deconstruction and reconstruction characteristic of contemporary societies under technological development. Nor does man, who is both the object and subject of this intoxicating adventure, escape—as is borne out in many ways by contemporary biomedical practices and examined by bioethical questioning. The current explosion of ethical questions could be tied to the kind of flawed premises you point out in the mechanistic theory, or it could indicate a paradigmatic shift favoring a plurality of views of life.

The fate of vitalism

IKEDA • Probably both. But it is time to look at another historically important view of life: vitalism. This is the very old idea that life results from a unique principle distinct from matter. The theory varies depending on whether vitality, or the *anima*, is considered the basic essence of life, or its structure, or its function. When applied in terms of structure or function, vitalism approaches an organic theory, a theory that distinguishes living beings from other systems of matter.

BOURGEAULT • To situate life and understand the living being, vitalism refers to another paradigm. In the living being, the "vital principle" struggles against laws of physics regarded as threats to or constraints on life. Vitalists believe that a force or principle of life—the vital principle—permits the body to remain in the physical world without being corrupted. At the beginning of the eighteenth century, Georg-Ernst Stahl (1660–1734) saw in the spiritual soul just such a principle of life and promise of incorruptibility.

IKEDA • Stahl is well known for his phlogiston theory. I believe "phlogiston" is derived from the Greek word for flammability or combustibility. The phlogiston theory was related to the vitalists' *anima* or vital principle. It is therefore understandable that, when Antoine L. Lavoisier (1743–94), the father of modern chemistry, refuted the phlogiston theory, the idea of the imperishable anima too declined.

BOURGEAULT • Vitalism was a major element of Stahl's medico-philosophical work, advanced as a reaction against mechanism. The more moderate Barthez (1734–1806), Bordeu (1722–76), and Bichat (1771–1802)—the most famous advocates of vitalism—attempted to understand and to help others understand the nature and functioning modes of a truly vital principle (at least analogically similar to the force of attraction and gravity defined by Newton). This force, though not subject to the laws of physics, was considered distinct from the spiritual soul. Vitalism enjoyed favor in European scientific circles during the second half of the eighteenth and especially at the beginning of the nineteenth century. But neither Bichat nor any of the others succeeded in constructing a modern vitalist physiology that could have been a counterpart to Newtonian physics. That is why vitalism has hardly any adherents today.

Mechanistic and vitalist views are no longer the only possibilities

IKEDA • Even though the phenomenon of life constitutes a unique fact, we are well advised to recognize a plurality of approaches to it. When we realize, as you point out, that views of life vary from epoch to epoch and from society to society, there is no reason to adhere to any one standardized view.

BOURGEAULT • Greco-Roman and Judeo-Christian traditions have resulted in a certain way of looking at things, legitimizing human dominion over life and the material universe. It is partly thanks to the mechanistic vision that what we call Western civilization emerged.

Then, little by little, scientific discoveries evoked the complex play of interdependencies and ineluctable solidarities among all living beings, paving the way for another vision. Here I would like to mention two other books, both testimonies to a paradigm shift, that have influenced the development of my own thought on this subject: *The Possible and the Actual*[16] by François Jacob and *Order out of Chaos: Man's New Dialogue with Nature*[17] by Ilya Prigogine and Isabelle Stengers. From the first, I learned how the abounding diversity of living beings is caught up in the same game of life. The second taught me how scientific development brings about changes in the relationship between human beings and other living creatures—and on a larger scale with nature and the cosmos—that orient science in new directions and provoke its metamorphosis.

IKEDA • These books seem to go beyond simple mechanistic arguments.

BOURGEAULT • Yes, they certainly do. The vision of life and its origins that you quite justly call materialist does not seem to me to be necessarily reductionist. Bearing in mind what we have already observed, I think that it first and foremost tries to account for hidden relationships that, beyond the obvious ruptures, assure continuity between matter and life. We are not compelled to choose between the mechanism of Descartes—and his biology inspired by Galileo's physics—and the vitalism of Bordeu or Bichat. Between the reductionist vision of life—with its well-oiled mechanics and its laws—and a vision that would snatch life from membership in the material realm and from the influence of the laws of physics and chemistry. As you were saying earlier, there are many subtle nuances in these two major currents of thought—mechanism and vitalism.

Toward a subjective, humanizing concept of life

IKEDA • On that point I agree with you entirely. Buddhism teaches that a profound understanding of the distinctive human characteristic of "self-awareness" helps us establish our own subjective views of life. As I have already mentioned, the theory of the nine consciousnesses,

16. François Jacob. *The Possible and the Actual.* Seattle: University of Washington Press. 1994.

17. Ilya Prigogine and Isabelle Stengers. *Order out of Chaos: Man's New Dialogue with Nature.* New York: Random House. 1984.

coupled with the concept of the five components, provides the basis for the Buddhist view of life.

The fifth component, or consciousness, gives birth to the components of perception, conception and volition and is where "humanity" begins. In grasping the profundity of the fifth component, we become conscious of ourselves. This state of self-awareness corresponds to the sixth of the nine consciousnesses and leads to the seventh consciousness, which enables us to contact the interior spiritual world. The seventh consciousness is the basis of the reflective, introspective self. It is constantly vulnerable to greed, conceit, and bitterness and so on, and it is here that we distinguish good from evil. If we can overcome our evil thoughts and inclinations at this level, we can radiate wisdom and reason. But how can such evil thought be overcome? The power is found in the still deeper eighth or *alaya* consciousness. There the self is one with the environment and, assimilating past experiences, it orients itself toward the future. In Buddhist terms, this consciousness is called the storehouse, and it contains all good and bad karma.

When the self is fused with the cosmos, with cosmic life, it attains the ninth consciousness, the pure, fundamental consciousness which is the ultimate source of energy for reinforcing good karma.

In this way, Buddhism explains how a "subjective perception" of life can evolve and transform. This is a major philosophic contribution.

BOURGEAULT • Personally, what I retain from debates between mechanists and vitalists is that there is no life except in living and that the understanding human beings can have of life depends on their constantly renewed experience of it. It is human beings who, aware of this experience, give meaning to life. Consequently, we can understand life only in reference to the contexts and categories of a social construct that reflects the developments of life in society.

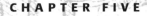

CHAPTER FIVE

DAWN OF
THE CENTURY OF LIFE

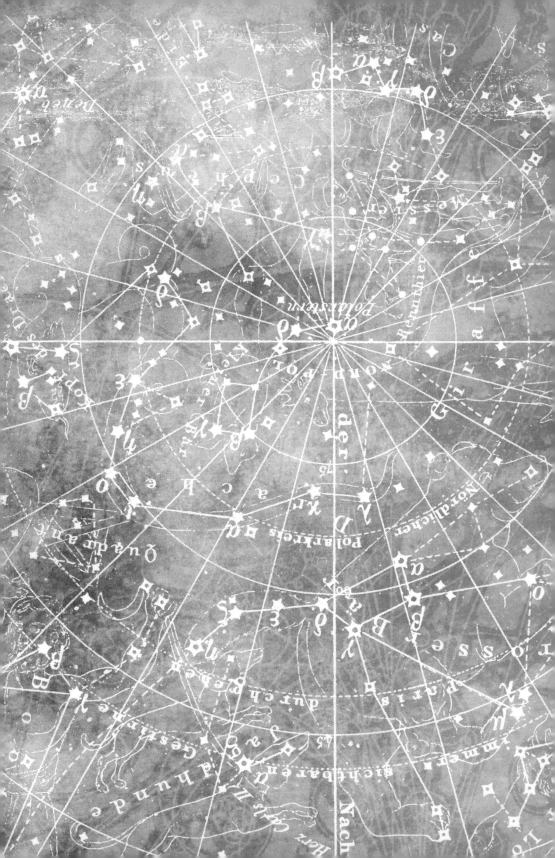

1. Pathology of our Time

The end of universal values

IKEDA • At the end of the twentieth century, dramatic changes unimaginable during the Cold War occurred in the world. With unexpected speed, the two Germanys were reunited. Strategic nuclear weapons belonging to both Cold War blocs were dismantled.

However, even in the wake of the democratization of the countries of Eastern Europe, problems abound. Ethnic conflicts in the former Yugoslavia are just one example. The serious economic crises in Asia and other parts of the world in the past few years are another symptom of the menacing clouds on humanity's horizons. I cannot help thinking our world is gravely ill.

BOURGEAULT • Yes, new chasms are opening up everywhere in our societies. Our dreams of solidarity and peace have been smothered in a thousand ways. For a time, we thought we had consigned the racism of Nazi Germany to the nightmares of the past. But the collapse of the Soviet Union revived the old demons—asleep but not gone—of interethnic rivalries. Blow by blow, we witnessed ethnic cleansing in Rwanda and the former Yugoslavia.

IKEDA • The situation is tragic. We have lost the universal values that go beyond ethnicity. Never has it been more essential to transcend ethnic, religious, and cultural differences and think in terms of the whole human race.

BOURGEAULT • In Europe and particularly in France, the fear of fundamentalist Islam simultaneously demonstrates and conceals resistance to social acceptance of ethnic, cultural, and religious diversity. What are things like in Japan in this connection?

IKEDA • Ever since the restoration of Meiji in 1868, Japan has consistently pursued a policy of assimilating ethnic minorities like the Ainu and other tribes in the northern part of the country. The rich Ryukyu culture of Okinawa, too, has been Japanized over the centuries. The ruling government before and during World War II extended such policies throughout the Japanese empire, to Korea, Taiwan, and the islands of the South Pacific.

In a sense, Japan was following the example of European colonial powers, which considered Asians and Africans "backward" and equated the introduction of their own cultures with enlightenment and development. The Japanese assimilation policy went too far, however, and refused to countenance even the ethnic diversity of local cultures.

The discriminatory attitude, long maintained in modern times, still persists among the Japanese today. The Japanese people have often taken a suspicious, contemptuous view of outside workers from Asia and Central and South America who come to the more prosperous Japan to work.

BOURGEAULT • In Canada, the land of immigrants (from France, and then Britain, and eventually pretty well everywhere: Italy, Spain, Portugal, China and India, Eastern Europe, the Caribbean, Latin America, and Africa . . .), demographic diversity is more evident in big cities like Vancouver, Toronto, and Montreal. But the dynamics of marginalization—if not exactly exclusion—are at work, resulting in ghettoes and misunderstanding.

IKEDA • Immigrants tend to congregate in ethnic enclaves, to live in the same neighborhoods, because they depend on their friends and families, because they are freshly arrived and because they share more or less the same economic circumstances. The result, however, is that their communities tend to fall victim to hostility and discrimination from other neighborhoods.

BOURGEAULT • We tend to blame "others" for our ills, especially for violence. They are not like us. But we forget that we ourselves are a composite of many different elements.

IKEDA • "A composite of different elements" is just another way of saying "rich diversity" for those who choose to see this reality in a positive light.

BOURGEAULT • To repeat what we have already said, life's developments are the result of encounters and exchanges that fulfill its precondition of diversity. Paradoxically, although exclusionist practices—sometimes as radical as ethnic cleansing—are rife in many regions, concern for threatened species stimulates us to try to protect plant and animal genetic diversity.

IKEDA • Yes. In the natural environment, protecting biological genetic diversity is considered important. Surely we ought to address the issue of protecting individual cultural diversity in our socio-cultural environment, too.

BOURGEAULT • Reminiscent of the economic order, a dynamic of competition—a struggle to the end tending to exclude others—is at work in our societies, leaving its mark on social developments and the political order.

IKEDA • We require a fundamental change. We must regard immigrants and citizens from other countries not as outsiders, but as our fellows. To see differences as a positive sign of diversity, we need the fundamental conviction that "we're all human." Establishing this as a basic tenet means adopting all humankind as our standard.

Protagoras (ca. 485–ca. 410 BCE) said, "Man is the measure of all things." His statement is generally dismissed as relativistic and sophist, but I believe it reveals insight into the profound truth that the only way to accommodate diverse value criteria is to make humanity the standard of judgment. The sole prescription for the world's malaise is profound love and concern for humanity itself.

Poverty and social health

BOURGEAULT • If the health of societies, like the health of individuals, depends on the effort made to re-establish equilibrium and harmony after ruptures and imbalances, we must admit that our societies are sick. Even gravely ill, as you say. Persistent poverty is a sign, or a symptom, of grave social malady.

IKEDA • In recent years, the economic gap between the industrialized North and the developing South has been widening, in spite of efforts to close it. While many people in the developing nations have neither roofs over their heads nor food to eat, in the industrialized nations, people consume far too many calories and pollute the environment by squandering energy sources.

BOURGEAULT • We hoped—and sometimes promised—that the industrial and technological developments of the twentieth century would be the source of wealth and well-being for everybody. We have to accept the evidence that such has not been the case. The century of technological prowess that brought historically unprecedented riches to some has consigned increasingly growing masses of humanity to marginalization and exclusion.

IKEDA • Many developing nations have tried to encourage industry and free themselves from poverty. But their efforts have been defeated by serious infrastructural deficiencies—lack of power generators, water-works, railways, roads and other infrastructure necessary for industrial society.

BOURGEAULT • As you point out, poverty is inseparably linked to the health of populations and societies. Numerous studies have established the correlation between poverty and sickness, between poverty and reduced life expectancy. And of course between poverty and reduced quality of life.

IKEDA • Not to mention the vicious circle of poor sanitary conditions and high birth and infant-mortality rates. When survival is precarious, people tend to produce more offspring. Then, when sanitary conditions improve faster than families manage to adjust their priorities, the result is often a demographic explosion that destroys any economic gains made.

BOURGEAULT • Although technological development makes imbalances more blatant and poverty more scandalous, it is not the cause of all the evils we observe.

The widening gap between rich and poor in industrialized countries

IKEDA • Very true. The material poverty of the developing countries is grave. For their part, the industrialized nations face a serious state of spiritual impoverishment glaringly revealed in growing drug abuse, juvenile delinquency, violence and crime. Although the industrialized nations have achieved great material wealth, the lowest strata of these societies have been left out. Worse yet, the disparities between the rich and the poor seem to have widened lately and become insurmountable.

BOURGEAULT • In Montreal, people living in the affluent, upper-crust Westmount neighborhood, on the west side of a hill proudly dubbed Mount Royal, enjoy a life expectancy, health status, and quality of life (real access to education, information, culture, etc.) that their fellow citizens at the foot of the mountain can only dream about.

IKEDA • Because the poor have no access to the social ladder, more and more young people are drifting emotionally and falling into a goal-less way of life, as if they were spiritually dried out. This "desertification of the soul" leaves them with no ambition in life other than to seek comfort and immediate pleasure. We have a "me" generation of beings unable to think of anything other than the immediate satisfaction of personal desires and totally disinterested in social issues. Our societies seem incapable of providing goals they can strive for.

BOURGEAULT • I find especially striking the gap between the well-off and the society's rejects, even in rich countries. In Canada's colossal neighbor, the United States, for example, social programs that are clearly inadequate, if not simply nonexistent, deprive large strata of the population of their share of the collective wealth of a nation that nonetheless boasts of staying in the first rank of international economic competition.

IKEDA • True. While poverty is a major problem for the industrialized nations, we must recognize that the developing nations face a material crisis, and the crisis of the industrialized nations is spiritual. One way or another, the whole world is plagued by extreme imbalance.

BOURGEAULT • The truly scandalous gap between industrialized and developing nations takes the form of exploitation of the poor by the rich for their own profit. Despite efforts to close this gap in recent decades, it has become more marked.

A new approach to economic assistance

IKEDA • For the moment, the first step is to launch an international campaign to better mobilize the aid that can help pull developing countries from their economic crises. Money and goods alone will be insufficient. Technological and cultural contributions—like education to raise literacy levels—are essential to putting the developing nations on the course of independent economic growth. Of course, economic development also demands a sufficient material basis, including industrial infrastructure.

For their part, industrialized nations must no longer be allowed to prosper by sacrificing the developing nations. Several of these richer countries, having greatly profited from the developing nations, have suddenly found themselves in economic difficulties. It is imperative that the industrialized nations reflect on what they have done and make restitution for their past actions and work to build a world of mutual prosperity.

BOURGEAULT • I wholeheartedly agree with your diagnosis. The material wealth of some to the detriment of others seems to be accompanied by an impoverishment of the spirituality that, over the centuries in diverse traditions, advocated and maintained compassion and solidarity—that is, sharing.

IKEDA • In our societies today we are witnessing a burgeoning protectionism, the preservation of the acquired rights of the privileged classes. This is a dangerous tendency, a nefarious type of conservatism.

BOURGEAULT • A friend once remarked to me, a few years ago, that those who become conservative are usually those with something to conserve! No doubt wealth could be and should be shared rather than hoarded. This probably explains why the prophets were constantly calling for compassion and sharing.

IKEDA • No doubt. Major religions like Buddhism and Christianity all teach compassion and love for all people and encourage practical expressions of benevolence and caring.

BOURGEAULT • Yes, but usually the poor have understood the words of prophets better than the rich.

IKEDA • Yes, the poorer they are, the more people are inclined to help each other. History abounds with instances of the downfall of the arrogant rich. Those of us who live in the rich countries should reflect deeply on this historical truism. No one can live without the support of other human beings. We must always keep this in mind and be grateful. Buddhism uses the expression "indebted to all sentient beings" to encourage people to feel grateful for the support, both tangible and intangible, we get from others.

BOURGEAULT • The thing that is new and specific to our own time is the persistence of poverty in societies that have the power to reduce it substantially or even to eliminate it.

IKEDA • Even though foreign aid programs contribute considerable sums to developing countries, the fate of the people of the beneficiary countries does not seem to have improved.

BOURGEAULT • An economist recently proposed the imposition of a tax—a mere 0.01%—on the cross-border financial exchanges that seem to control everything today. This tax would impoverish no one and, if I follow the reasoning correctly, would bring annual returns of more than US$100 billion. Such an amount would feed immense numbers of undernourished people, care for and cure them, educate them, train them, and provide them with access to global knowledge.

IKEDA • An excellent idea. A fraction of the great wealth accumulated in the hands of a few can save hundreds of millions of lives in the world. Professor Amartya Sen (1933–) from India received the first Nobel Prize for economics in 1998, for his "economics of poverty," the basic premise of which is saving the poor and weak. Instead of the money games of the rich, Professor Sen's thesis sheds ethical light on an economic activity designed to enrich the poor.

Because domestic conditions in donor nations can destabilize economic assistance, we must re-examine the current system of nation-to-nation aid. Much more could be accomplished if impartial international organizations like the United Nations and the World Bank were given greater resources and invested with the necessary authority to set up effective aid systems.

Swords into ploughshares

BOURGEAULT · Some years ago, under the leadership of Mrs. Gro Harlem Brundtland (1939–), the United Nations World Commission on Environment and Development came to similar conclusions and recommended that the sums currently used for armament be devoted to the battle against poverty and the protection of the environment.

IKEDA · I am quite familiar with the UN commission and Mrs. Brundtland. When Soka Gakkai International held its "War and Peace" exhibition in Oslo in 1991, we received a message from Mrs. Brundtland, who was Norwegian prime minister at the time. She thought highly of our efforts to promote grassroots awareness of the problems of peace and the environment and said she was happy to have found a good partner in SGI.

Our Common Future, the report that the World Commission on Environment and Development published in 1987, clearly shows how these planetary issues are closely interrelated. The concept of sustainable development elucidated in the document embraces development, the struggle against poverty and environmental protection and preservation.

BOURGEAULT · Rich nations consider UN peace-keeping missions too expensive. Yet wars supported by arms manufacturers, respected people in those same rich nations, make such missions necessary. Incontrovertibly, however, the arms industry provides very fertile ground for the development of highly advanced technologies. We are faced with something of a paradox.

IKEDA · To be sure, a wide gap separates reality from the ideal. This is all the more reason for us to set our ideals even higher. For example, a group of scholars tried to demonstrate that peace, not war, pays off. I respect these people and I appreciate their efforts to start with the reality and point out concrete ways to attain the ideal. On the other hand, some people set an ideal without thought of how it might be attained. Such an attitude seems unrealistic. As Mahatma Gandhi said, a good thing moves with the speed of a snail.

BOURGEAULT • That is why at the international level, the UN is paralyzed and its programs are often unproductive. With growing frequency, people criticize the UN for ineffectiveness, but by refusing to give the organization the means to act, they compel it to be ineffective. I said this ten years ago when I was chairman of the Canadian UNESCO Commission. It was at this time that the United States withdrew from this great agency under the pretext of its mismanagement (that is to say, management inspired by precepts other than the ones championed by the United States!) and inefficacious actions. UNESCO was then experiencing financial difficulties caused by the failure of many member nations, including the United States, to pay their dues. This has recently become especially glaring in connection with UN peace-restoration and peace-keeping missions, which have been delayed by the reluctance of member nations, especially the richest, to collaborate. Those same member nations always later lament the failure to prevent crises or intervene in them before it was too late.

IKEDA • Achieving just goals demands just means, not merely the immediate expedient. As I said earlier, in the oriental tradition, the best doctor is the one who prevents the disease, not the one who cures it. The same thing applies to people who wish to cure society.

Changing worldly desires to wisdom and enlightenment

BOURGEAULT • Rereading the section of the three temptations of Christ in Dostoyevsky's (1821–81) *The Brothers Karamazov* a few years ago stimulated my reflections on these questions. The author presents a living Jesus undergoing three experiences that make up the fabric of all human existence. The French philosopher Paul Ricoeur (1913–) calls them the three dynamics of a triple appetite: possession, worth, and power. The dynamic of possession can be experienced either as accumulating and monopolizing or exchanging, giving, and sharing. The dynamic of worth can either follow the tangent of self-actualization in the ceaseless search for prestige or seek encounters with others.

The dynamic of power can contribute to domination and subjugation or to mutual aid in solidarity and recognized interdependence. I am sure that similar orientations are to be found in Buddhism.

IKEDA • "The three dynamics of a triple appetite" . . . This perceptive expression reveals the essence of human desires. Buddhism does have a similar concept. The three desires you spoke of signify a kind of self-aggrandizement. In other words, they represent the self-love that seeks to enlarge the ego and all its appurtenances. Buddhism perceives these desires or illusions as sources of physical and spiritual suffering, and as hindrances to the quest for enlightenment.

Mahayana Buddhism teaches that Buddhahood can be attained, not by extinguishing earthly desires and illusions, but by using them as energy to create happiness for oneself and others. This is expressed in the doctrine "earthly desires are enlightenment." In other words, desires must first exist; then, correctly mastered and channeled desires can become a source of energy to create happiness for both the self and others.

"Burn the kindling of earthly desires," teaches Nichiren, "and warm yourself at the fire of wisdom and enlightenment." Without desire (the kindling), we cannot transform reality into the wisdom (the warmth and light of the fire) that contributes to the happiness of others. If we own nothing ourselves, we have nothing to share. The important thing is the resolve to transform the firewood of desire into the flame of wisdom.

BOURGEAULT • Of course we must *have* in order to be able to give or share. Of course we must be appreciated and self-actualized to develop the self-confidence that enables us to acknowledge the other. Of course we must master our own lives and environments to establish relations of mutual aid and solidarity. But we can easily observe something entirely different in current individual and collective behavior. Savage economic competition at the international level strives to eliminate competitors. Talk about promoting excellence ultimately plays into the hands of advocates of domination and exploitation of the poor and weak by the rich and strong, legitimizing their point of view.

Does this mean that society and humanity are sick? The health of societies, like that of all humanity and of individual human beings, depends not on the absence of sickness, but on the constant effort to re-establish balance. In spite of our much-touted technological feats and commercial success, poverty is gaining ground. It affects the young and the old most. Gravest of all, it seems to me, is that this reality is ascribed more to fatality than to responsibility. It stands to reason that we can change nothing as long as we believe in fatalism, which I refuse to adopt.

IKEDA • We must neither avert our eyes from harsh realities nor turn a deaf ear to the agonized voices of the real world. We must keep our hearts and minds open to the suffering of others and accept it as if it were our own. I myself am determined to take a personal concern in all human affairs because this is the meaning of Buddhist empathy and compassion, the bodhisattva way. Buddhism seeks to change the destiny of the world. Essentially it teaches that, since fate results from our own acts, our own acts can transform fate. This is the meaning of the SGI "human revolution" movement.

BOURGEAULT • It is not true that we are impotent. We have the knowledge and the technological and financial means to change things—I almost said "to change the world." But it is difficult, when we are among the most privileged members of a system, to really want to change it.

IKEDA • But we must overcome that difficulty by concentrating on cultivating the inner human being. The problems that have arisen as a result of industrial development are rooted, I believe, in the scientific and technological civilization of modern times, which encourages the accumulation of materials goods and the immediate satisfaction of desire.

For most of history, humanity was at the mercy of the generosity of the laws of nature. It is only with the most recent technological revolutions that we have begun to develop the natural environment and modify it in ways that improve our own standard of living. We were quick to believe that the natural world existed to be controlled and endlessly exploited for our benefit. Today we understand that this vision of nature was an important factor in the emergence of a set of interrelated global problems—pollution, environmental destruction, and so on—that comprise the biggest challenge human civilization has ever faced.

People in all fields of human endeavor must question their goals. We must use our wisdom for the sake of all humanity.

BOURGEAULT • Even though technological development makes imbalance more glaring and poverty more scandalous, it is not the sole cause of the ills we see around us.

IKEDA • True. After all, we are the ones who create and employ technology. So the only choice left to us is to transform humans themselves, to create a new kind of person. This is the key to the spiritual crisis in industrialized societies. Our sole recourse is to develop individuals worthy of the task of building a new century of hope. Otherwise the world will be filled with more and more people who care little about the suffering of their fellow humans and who show themselves less and less inclined to reach out a hand to a neighbour in distress.

2. Goals of Education

Value-creating education for the well-being of humans

IKEDA • Our conversation has led us naturally to the vast subject of education: how can we develop generous individuals who care for their fellow beings? Education presents an immense challenge for our long-term future. I have always believed, even when I was a young man, that education was among the most noble vocations.

BOURGEAULT • If I remember correctly, Soka Gakkai came into being as a group of educators determined to devote themselves to the well-being of individuals, communities, and all humanity.

IKEDA • It is true that education is almost meaningless unless it contributes to the happiness of individuals and, by extension, humanity in general. Tsunesaburo Makiguchi, originator of the theory of value-creating education, insisted that the happiness of children is of primary importance.

Both the first and second presidents of Soka Gakkai believed firmly that the goal of education must be to create joy and happiness in everyday life. As their successor, I too am completely devoted to this goal. I want to see all people challenge the four sufferings, cultivate their physical and spiritual strength, blaze their own trails to happiness, and prepare themselves to triumph over all the adversities they will have to face during their lives.

To make this great dream a reality, I have founded the Soka schools and Soka University, as institutions where President Makiguchi's value-creating educational theory can be put into practice.

Dr. Simard and Dr. Bourgeault, you have both also been involved for a long time in the education of young men and women. What kind of education can help inspire an ideal life—overcoming the four sufferings and pursuing the well-being of others and of humanity in general?

Education and solidarity

BOURGEAULT · Drawing on the categories proposed by Marcel Lesne some fifteen years ago, I would distinguish three models of pedagogy corresponding to three visions of education and relationships between teacher and student—or, as they say today, learner. The first model categorizes education as the transmission of already established knowledge. This is an apprenticeship defined as assimilation and repetition. The accent is put squarely on established, apparently immutable knowledge.

IKEDA · Because it over-emphasizes the importance of knowledge, Japanese education turns out students incapable of analyzing and applying what they learn. The knowledge that they memorized is of no use to them when they find themselves in trouble.

Another weakness of an education predicated entirely on knowledge is the decline of ethics and altruism among students. Instead of regarding their fellow students as friends, they think of them as competitors who must be defeated in the race for diplomas and admission to the top universities. This kind of education will probably produce heartless people—albeit very well informed and professionally successful—who care nothing for others.

BOURGEAULT · This is what Paulo Freire (1921–97) calls the banker's idea of knowledge and education. Perhaps, too, schools often encourage the accumulation of fragmented, juxtaposed knowledge instead of considering connections among realities.

At the center of the second of my two models is the learner as an autonomous subject responsible for his or her own learning. To take the initiative in developing their knowledge, the learners approach each subject on the basis of personal experience, tastes, and interests. The system seeks to make the students capable of enunciating their own experiences in clear language, of appropriating and digesting dispensed knowledge, and of integrating it with their own store of knowledge.

As an example, I remember my own first year of teaching. One of the students in the group, who had failed the year before, seemed totally unable to do literary analysis. Indeed he was convinced he could not. I was teaching theater at the time and was in charge of a dramatic-arts studio. I knew he was interested in photography and architecture so, perhaps out of intuition or as a challenge, I instructed him to read the text of the play we were going to present the following semester and to make suggestions about the settings. Ten days later, he came back with a superb scale model and began explaining and justifying his proposals based on an analysis of the text that he had carried out without even realizing it.

IKEDA • No doubt this method of assimilating knowledge spontaneously through practical experience has its advantages, but it could lead to egoism, especially if the learner has no chance to cultivate a sense of ethics.

BOURGEAULT • That is true. My third model stresses the relationship between the teacher and the learner and strives to develop a critical spirit by contextualizing knowledge and revealing its connections with the society that generated it. Knowledge is never neutral. Created in relation to social conflict and often reflecting the viewpoint of the dominant group, knowledge helps maintain the domination of that group over others. This kind of teaching is harder for the teacher than for the learner (we can only hope that the teacher is a learner, too). It also seems more likely to develop what I would call a civic conscience—at the local, national, and even global level—and to prepare people to act as responsible citizens in pluralist societies.

Shakyamuni the teacher

IKEDA • Your third model reminds me of the way Shakyamuni taught. Shakyamuni lived among the people plunged into the torment of the four sufferings and so developed empathy. Out of compassion he taught them how to overcome their hardships. He gave the sick wisdom and courage to fight against their illnesses. He sometimes nursed them himself. He and his disciple Ananda bathed them and made their beds while listening to their troubles, giving them advice, and instructing them in Buddhist teachings.

Shakyamuni always adapted his teachings to the understanding of his listeners. His pedagogical method is often compared to a good medical treatment, always dictated in response to the patient's specific symptoms. Your third teaching model has something in common with Shakyamuni's philosophy.

SIMARD • Your description of Shakyamuni's teaching method reminds me of Socratic dialectic. In the Athens of Socrates' day, most teachers were content simply to transmit received knowledge as if on a conveyor belt. They required their students to memorize the epics of Homer, which were interpreted in strictly predetermined ways. Socrates broke that mold by constantly asking his students questions. Each answer stimulated another question. Taking the maieutic method to its height, he helped his students think for themselves and mature intellectually. His dialogues were a very dynamic and effective teaching method.

IKEDA • As an illustration of the way Shakyamuni adjusted his teaching method to the situation, I might cite the story of Kisa Gotami who, in her grief, asked him to revive her recently deceased child.

SIMARD • What was his response?

IKEDA • He sent her around the village asking for mustard seeds. He said he would revive her child if she would bring him a mustard seed from a house whose family had never lost anyone to death.

SIMARD • But no house can ever be completely free from death.

IKEDA • Exactly. As she went frantically from house to house seeking one where no one had died, Kisa Gotami came to a deep realization of the inevitability of death for all living things. This enlightenment inspired in her the determination to overcome her own grief. Shakyamuni then taught her the truth of Buddhist law and invited her to join him in his quest to find ways to transcend life and death.

BOURGEAULT · In your 1990 speech at Peking University, which appears in *A New Humanism*,[1] you said that education is not just teaching or instructing. Education requires teachers to ask questions that lead students on the way to self-learning and growth.

IKEDA · Dr. S. Mohan (1930–), former supreme court justice of India, and Professor David W. Chappell (1940–), who teaches religion at the University of Hawaii at Manoa, both emphasize the importance of dialogue in education.

In a speech delivered in Osaka, Dr. Mohan said, "Education must not be control of students by teachers. It is not unilateral, but a teacher-student dialogue." Professor Chappell insists on the reciprocity of the pedagogical process. In other words, the teachers do not just teach the students, they also learn from them. Education is both giving and receiving. It is a two-way communication and an effort to bring the value out in everyone.

It seems to me that we cannot hope to stimulate the vitality, wisdom, courage and compassion needed to face the challenges of life and triumph over adversity except through fruitful dialogue between teacher and learner. Only then can knowledge take firm root in the learner's heart.

It is likely that in animated exchanges between teacher and learner, objective knowledge becomes living and useful and enables the learner to triumph over individual egoism.

Your three pedagogical models, Dr. Bourgeault, have counterparts in the Buddhist world view. The first model, centered on the assimilation of established knowledge, is similar to the World of Learning (*shomon*). These disciples of the Buddha listen to his sermons and work toward enlightenment.

The second model, with its objective of attaining knowledge through personal experience, corresponds to the World of Realization (*engaku*). At this stage, people perceive the links of causality in nature

---

1. Daisaku Ikeda. *A New Humanism*. New York: Weatherhill Inc. 1996.

and are awakened to the impermanence of all phenomena through their own observations and efforts.

The third model, focused on teacher/learner exchange, evokes the figure of the bodhisattva, whose deepest concern is the well-being of others. In consequence, what you called solidarity education leads the teacher and learner to the practice of the bodhisattva way. This pedagogical model helps people overcome the four sufferings and live for the good of humanity.

Teaching how to learn

IKEDA • Now that we have a good idea about what education should be, perhaps we could talk about the ideal teacher-student relationship in the light of what we understand as the university's mission.

SIMARD • Yes, that's an excellent way to move into our topic. In *The Idea of a University* (1873), Cardinal John Henry Newman (1801–90) presents the university as a secluded place where students wishing to learn encounter professors who guide them in the synthesis of knowledge and help them understand that the human factor is the most important element in all theories of culture, technology, and science. As the founder of Soka University, Mr. Ikeda, what is your reaction to the cardinal's view?

IKEDA • His idea of the university sets forth the ideal relationship between student and teacher. For students, the important thing is how to learn. Tsunesaburo Makiguchi insisted that teachers should impart, not mere information, but knowledge of how to learn.

SIMARD • Mr. Makiguchi was absolutely right. It is easy to see that he was an educator in the true sense of the word. The wisdom of his comments on learning can only grow more significant with the passing of time.

The ultimate aim of the educational mission is the complete development of the student as a responsible citizen and a future professional. At the university level, this development goes beyond the acquisition of immediately applicable knowledge and entails developing a capacity to reflect and consequently to act in such a way as to deepen the significance and usefulness of knowledge to the progress of the human spirit.

Teaching is an act of communication, perhaps the most ambiguous and unsettling of all. Professors act not only as communicators and experts in their fields, but also and more importantly as teachers and witnesses to scientific, intellectual, moral, social, and cultural values. They must accompany students in their evolution, adjust themselves to various training situations, intervene to facilitate understanding of pursued objectives, and demonstrate the real complementary nature of proposed educational actions. In a word, teachers must be there for the students and supervise them as they progress.

IKEDA • The goal is to develop not a fact-crammed mind but what Montaigne calls a well-seasoned mind.[2]

SIMARD • Achieving that means university professors must be more than specialists in their own fields and communicators of particular kinds of knowledge. They must also become models in ethical, social, and cultural spheres. Consequently, university professors are responsible for both the transmission of knowledge and the cultivation of scientists who have both open and critical spirits and who can show themselves capable of working to integrate their studies, their analyses, and the results of their intellectual efforts in an inclusive perspective.

Flexible spirit, sure judgment, and perseverance

SIMARD • Contrary to what is often thought, the important thing in science is as much the spirit that sustains the process as the end result. It is as much the openness to novelty, critical rigor, and submission to the unexpected—no matter how annoying—as the result itself—no matter how new and extraordinary. Scientists have long renounced the idea of an ultimate, tangible truth, the exact image of a reality just waiting to be unveiled. They now know they must be satisfied with the partial and the provisional. They realize that, in general, we have not really been looking for what we have found and have not always found what we were looking for. They know that, at every instant, a new way that must be explored opens up. From this arises the imperious necessity of a vast general culture.

---

2. Michel de Montaigne. *Essays*. Montreal: Pocketbooks. 1956.

In fact, modern science dates from the moment we began to substitute limited questions for general mythological or religious questions. Instead of asking how the universe was created, what matter is made of, and who gave birth to life, we started asking why a stone falls, how water circulates in a tube, and how species reproduce. This change in attitude and perception had amazing consequences. Whereas general questions got limited responses, limited questions led to increasingly general answers.

The same approach is valid today. This is the approach young student researchers who want a successful career in science must adopt. Researchers in the human and laboratory sciences must have certain important qualities. They must be able to judge when problems have become ripe for analysis. They must decide when it is time to explore unknown terrain and, in the light of new facts, return to questions already considered solved or unsolvable. To a large extent, an open spirit and sound judgment correspond to creativity and innovation in science. Promising talent is revealed by tendencies and aptitudes of this kind.

IKEDA • In any field of endeavor, perseverance is a necessary ingredient of success. But we need to know our goal and keep it in mind. The goal is the reason for persistence and the spur that stimulates perseverance.

For Buddhists, the most fundamental practice is to ceaselessly observe our own minds, elevate our goals and thereby raise our life condition. We believe that the principles and energy needed for self-improvement are to be found within ourselves. The goal of Buddhist practice is to activate and strengthen these innate qualities and enable every individual to lead a life worthy of humanity. The *Lotus Sutra* explains the three characteristics of the bodhisattva as the Robe of Forbearance, the Seat of Emptiness, and the Room of Compassion.[3]

The Robe of Forbearance stands for the unyielding determination to challenge and endure all hardships courageously. The Seat of Emptiness refers to the wisdom that understands the essential nature of all things and to a state of infinite flexibility as vast as the sky. The

3. *The Lotus Sutra*. Tr. Burton Watson. New York: Columbia University Press. 1993. Chapter 10.

Room of Compassion means a caring and empathetic attitude toward all people and the desire to find happiness with them.

These three qualities—determination, wisdom, and compassion—correspond almost perfectly with the idea of promising talent you were describing.

Dr. Simard, you mentioned Cardinal Newman's definition of the university. Along the same lines, I believe that respect for humanity is the basis for all knowledge and should be the starting point of education at every level. This is why Tsunesaburo Makiguchi held the well-being of students as the main goal of education.

The ultimate goal of education and research is the good of humankind. Learning is the means, humanity is the end. We must never reverse these priorities. Knowledge acquired through the search for truth must be put to use for humanity. Computers are capable of storing information and using it to analyze problems. But only human beings can determine how such information will be used. In the end, only humans know how to teach others how to grow in wisdom and sensitivity.

From this perspective, a university is a privileged place where teachers and students together shoulder the responsibility of ensuring the continuity and full flowering of the "human element."

The most precious jewel: The wisdom of the Buddha

IKEDA · Tsunesaburo Makiguchi once said "Teaching is the noblest art and the most difficult skill, and only the best, most devoted people can hope to succeed at it—because its subject is the precious jewel of life itself."

SIMARD · Mr. Makiguchi had the courage to demonstrate what a true educator should be like. Every good educational institution has teachers who appreciate the true objectives of education. If these teachers' educational philosophy is logically reflected in the curricula of the school, college, or university that employs them, that institution will distinguish itself.

IKEDA · Today schools in Brazil understand and practice Makiguchi's educational theories. And we hope others will follow suit. Makiguchi's reference to life as a gem is based on the *Lotus Sutra*, in which the compassionate wisdom of the Buddha is called the supreme jewel inherent in all people. The reason for the appearance of Shakyamuni Buddha in this world was to open the door of Buddha wisdom to all living beings, to show it to them, to cause them to awaken to it, and to induce them to enter its path.

In his quest to find ways to overcome the four sufferings, Shakyamuni concluded that every individual must awaken to the sacred infinite nature of human life. Because of this teaching, Shakyamuni was called the Teacher of heavenly and human beings (*shasta devanam ca manushanam*). Mr. Makiguchi particularly liked this teaching and wrote a commentary on it.

SIMARD • All this shows how great a teacher Makiguchi was. In active rapport with a teacher of his stature, students can learn how to attain their goals and come to understand the importance of evolving ethically and responsibly. I know from experience that scientists and scholars of the first order come from the ranks of gifted, curious, and hardworking students.

Incidentally, antiquity provides the best example of a teacher-student relationship in the case of Socrates, who was Plato's instructor in thought. In his turn, Plato taught Aristotle, who became the tutor of Alexander the Great. Closer to us might be cited the gratitude Pierre and Marie Curie felt for Professor Beckerel or the adulation of Pasteur's pupils.

3. The Mission of the University

Safeguarding academic freedom

SIMARD • We seem to have concluded that education promoting solidarity and exchange between teacher and student helps to overcome the four sufferings. Moreover, we have identified how applicable that model is to the bodhisattva way. In *The Idea of a University*, Newman relies on the following three traits to define the university: (1) An autonomous institution acting at the nerve center of society; (2) A place of truth, where people can explore the importance of political, economic, and cultural development; and (3) A place of investigation of the choices made by the community and the value system of society. What impression does Newman's proposal for an ideal university make on you? What conception do you have of the university of today?

IKEDA • Newman covers all the important points. The first has to do with the major human-rights issue of academic freedom. History offers numerous examples of governments abusing learning and research for political purposes—Nazi Germany and the Soviet Union under Stalin (1879–1953), for instance. And in Japan, in connection with AIDS contracted from contaminated blood products, some official research workers issued data favorable to the interests of the pharmaceutical industry.

SIMARD • "Publish or perish!" For many years, this has been the prevailing mentality in academia and among researchers. For whatever purpose, this mindset breeds excessive competition that can lead to dishonesty and falsification of data and facts. Sadly, innumerable examples of such behavior tarnish the name of science and testify to intolerance, greed, and division at the very heart of the academic community.

It is high time for researchers—especially those in university employ—to examine their own deeper motivations. Are they carrying out research to promote knowledge of natural phenomena or for their own benefit and advancement? Is scientific publication a means of communicating discoveries or an exercise destined solely to ensure their own professional survival? Is the peer-review system an honest mechanism of evaluation or a reflection of a merciless struggle to ensure the survival of a school, a discipline, or even a university? Is scientific research justified as a human activity essential to enriching human knowledge about our environment or is it only a tool of transient utility?

IKEDA • It is a matter of the scientist's conscience. The researcher who loses sight of the search for truth and acts out of selfish interest also loses sight of his or her own obligation to society and humanity.

Universities must ensure the right to conduct research and publish findings according to the dictates of the scholar's own conscience, independent of political or economic considerations. This is why I advocate the establishment of education as a fourth governmental branch independent of the executive, judicial, and legislative branches. The integrity and credibility of the world of knowledge depend above all on the freedom of researchers to study, think and publish based only on their own conscience.

SIMARD • Precisely. That is why I should like to see all university graduates equip themselves with the following qualifications and capabilities. (1) Knowledge of the basic principles and methodology of their field; (2) An awareness of the limitations of their own field and receptivity to discoveries and methods in other fields; (3) A keenly critical spirit; (4) The ability to pursue independent study to enlarge and deepen their knowledge and understanding; (5) The ability to communicate ideas effectively and accurately; and (6) A sense of professional ethics.

IKEDA • You have covered all the conditions needed for a scientist or researcher. Graduates of higher institutes of learning are expected to be well informed in their own fields of specialization, but they should not gloat over their own knowledge. True scientists are always ready to improve and lend a humble ear to those in other fields. At the same time, they must be prepared to defend their own ethical views and refine their human nature.

This is the real heart of the question, don't you think? Ethics and education are inseparable insofar as they exert an enormous influence on the kind of lives people lead and the kind of happiness they can attain. The skills of the researcher that you just summed up are absolutely necessary for the preservation of liberty and, by extension, the integrity of the university.

Harmonizing the university's mission and society's needs

SIMARD • How do you react to Cardinal Newman's second point in *The Idea of a University*?

IKEDA • I believe it defines the essential role of the university in its search for truth. The university's role is to constantly reappraise politics, economics, and culture, which constitute the basic framework of human endeavor. The university and learning itself are founded on this undertaking.

SIMARD · Traditionally, the mission of the university has been to create and disseminate knowledge considered desirable in the society it is part of. Research and teaching have been the two wheels of the vehicle performing this double function.

While fulfilling this essential mission, the university must remain in close contact with the surrounding society in order to respond to its needs, understand the profile of new talents and new forms of knowledge, and develop and control new technologies to understand and exploit their potential. Big businesses devote significant sums to the professional training of their personnel and to research and development. This means they either are or ultimately will be natural partners of the university. Small businesses have even greater need of university resources because they can afford to devote much less money to the same cause. They are better able to fulfill their research and training responsibilities if they enter into a partnership with the university. All businesses large and small obviously rely on young university graduates for revitalization. Moreover, synergy between the university and business, between the professional world and its surrounding collectivities, is necessary not only to the preparation of the elite of tomorrow, but also to a critical appraisal of the choices society makes on the basis of new technologies and social evolution.

IKEDA · The production of knowledge in institutes of higher learning and research provides a basis for investigating the meaning of cultural, political, and economic development.

SIMARD · In addition to its traditional mission, the university now faces new social and ethical issues engendered by progress in high technology. Should we give priority to development or to the environment? Conflicts arise between civil rights and civil duties. These new issues seriously challenge established values.

All university graduates and holders of advanced degrees must have the capacity to think independently about complex problems and to form opinions in accordance with their own consciences. I hope they will each individually be able to equip themselves with what Montaigne called a well-seasoned mind. I am firmly convinced that a university must provide the means to acquire not only specialized knowledge, but also a minimal understanding of culture.

IKEDA • In April 1998, I had the opportunity to speak with Dr. Pan Yunhe (1946–), president of Zhejian University in China. Dr. Pan is an electronics specialist familiarly known as "Mr. Computer." He has given a great deal of thought to the idea of education in general and he expressed ideas that coincide exactly with yours. For instance, he insists that, although specialist knowledge is a must, students must acquire broader cultivation as well.

SIMARD • I completely agree with Dr. Pan. Educated people of our time must stay up-to-date by acquiring all sorts of knowledge and information in science and the humanities. We cannot expect to understand what is going on in the world unless we equip ourselves with basic knowledge on a wide range of subjects.

IKEDA • Tragically, just when Japan is facing so many serious problems, the country currently lacks leaders capable of providing such broad cultivation.

Interaction with society

SIMARD • What do you think about the third point in Cardinal Newman's definition of a university?

IKEDA • If I understand correctly, the third point has to do with the interaction of the university with society through its contributions as a producer and distributor of knowledge. The university has the responsibility to be aware of current trends and forecast future trends to see how they stack up against what their research indicates about safety or harmful repercussions. At the first sign of danger or suggestion of an undesirable tendency, the university must put society on its guard. Likewise, it must encourage positive currents and developments that promise to be valuable.

SIMARD • It seems to me that an important university function today is to engage in large-scale dialogues with society. Until the present, rapid industrial and technological advance has been the hallmark of postmodern society. What is the role of science in such a society? University professors and researchers must find a sensible, acceptable answer to this critical question through uninterrupted, penetrating dialogue with the rest of society.

IKEDA • I believe you are saying that academics must not shut themselves up in ivory towers.

SIMARD • Exactly. Universities must become more sensitive to the needs of society than they are at present. They have an obligation to identify new talent and new forms of knowledge and to develop the kind of technology and know-how conducive to the full flowering of society.

IKEDA • Dynamic exchanges with real society have stimulated dramatic progress in learning during various periods of history: the age of Shakyamuni in India, the era of the Hundred Philosophers in China (ca. 500–221 BCE), and the Renaissance in Europe. The mutual enlightenment of the university and non-academic society encourages both social development and a re-examination of ethical values, accelerating the evolution of society.

SIMARD • To give a specific example, universities should institute ways of submitting conferences and seminars to constant critical examination to ensure they conform with changing social realities. Teachers must take care that progress in diverse areas does not render their course material passé. It is their professional duty to keep abreast of the latest discoveries, to develop innovative methods, to open unexplored research horizons, and to present their discoveries to students with the least possible delay. This imposes heavy demands on teachers to read huge numbers of articles and research reports. Nowadays, it is nearly unthinkable for professors, no matter what their specialty, to give the same course more than once.

IKEDA • In Japan, sadly, some scholars actually do use the same lecture notes, year in and year out, to the despair of their students. As you say, Dr. Simard, course material must be constantly updated to conform with and apply to reality.

The happiness and well-being of the students is the most important reason to do so. Mr. Makiguchi said that education is not supervision but affection. Teaching is a vocation and a sacred responsibility toward the future not only of students, but also of all humanity. Educators in all fields and administrators at all levels must never forget that they are involved in a very noble mission.

4. Ethical Aspects of Technoscientific Development

An ethic worthy of global issues

BOURGEAULT • The report *No Limits to Learning: Bridging the Human Gap*,[4] submitted to the Club of Rome in 1979, by James W. Botkin, Mahdi Elamndjira, and Mircea Malitza, clearly demonstrated the amplitude and urgency of the challenge posed by the constantly widening gap between the complexity of our problems—including peace and harmony among human beings, the habitability of the planet, and the earth's continued capacity to support life—and our ability to find appropriate solutions. The authors of the report cite a model of research imprisoned by narrow technoscientific rationality. But such a model is outmoded in the search for solutions to real problems.

IKEDA • I have been associated with the Club of Rome for many years. I published a dialogue with its founder, the late Dr. Aurelio Peccei (1908–84), on the topic of the complexity of the problems that threaten the survival of humankind.[5] I also held a series of talks with his successor, Dr. Diez Hochleitner. Humanity now confronts unprecedented problems that we cannot resolve unless we pool the wisdom of as many people as possible.

In the preceding pages, we have discussed the need for a new ethic to help us eradicate such difficulties as poverty and environmental destruction. The regulation and control of technology are important corollaries to this ethic. Recent dramatic advances in genetic engineering and manipulation, too, have given rise to serious ethical problems. It is important to remember that genetic engineering makes life itself the object of technology. This runs the danger of regarding life in terms of commodity values or production efficiency or as a mere physical entity or even a consumer product.

Diversity itself partly explains our marvel and veneration for living things. Individuality gives life its dignity. When commercial worth becomes the criterion, that dignity crumbles. To ensure that all fields

4. James W. Botkin *et al. No Limits to Learning: Bridging the Human Gap.* New York: Pergamon Press. 1979.

5. Aurelio Peccei and Daisaku Ikeda. *Before It Is Too Late.* ed. Richard L. Cage. Tokyo – New York – London: Kodansha International. 1984.

of scientific technology reflect sound ethical standards, we must revise our social and legal systems and exercise control over science and technology.

BOURGEAULT · In 1989, a group of experts meeting in Vancouver, at the initiative of UNESCO, urgently pressed for a long-term, united effort to ensure the survival of the planet. The *Vancouver Declaration* resulting from the meeting begins, "Survival of the planet has become of central and immediate concern. The present situation requires urgent measures in all sectors—scientific, cultural, economic, and political—and a greater sensitization of all mankind. We must make common cause with all people on earth against a common enemy: any action that threatens balance within our environment, or reduces our legacy to future generations."[6]

IKEDA · The question is *who* is to be responsible for the necessary social and legislative systems.

BOURGEAULT · The future of humanity and of life on our planet will depend on controlling technological development. What kind of control will be exercised? How will it be enforced? In this instance, ethical issues become political. The technocratic model, which involves only experts and the initiated, is always attractive because it gives an appearance of prompt effectiveness. As I have said, however, this model has turned out to be ineffective. In democratic societies, social control assumes that the people responsible for developing and utilizing new technologies will be accountable to the general citizenry. It also assumes that the citizenry will be represented in decision-making organizations and will participate in debate leading to important decisions that ultimately affect the whole world.

The need for debate

IKEDA · The technological and scientific achievements of the past hundred years have exerted unprecedented influence on human society. Just think about how they have transformed the industrial structure,

---

6. Joint UNESCO – Canadian UNESCO Commission publication. Report on the conference "Symposium on Science and Culture for the 21st Century: Agenda for Survival." Vancouver, September 10–15, 1989.

for example, or communications and information processing systems. Perhaps we should call the twentieth century the "age of techno-scientific civilization."

On the negative side, these developments have generated serious problems like environmental destruction and human alienation. Despite this—believing that if science continues to proceed as it has been, it will one day find an answer for everything—humanity seems to have given it tacit approval to pursue its development according to its own internal logic.

Throughout the twentieth century, science was a great experiment. But the time has come to deeply reflect and seriously debate whether it has truly helped us realize the ideals of human happiness and global peace.

BOURGEAULT • Like you, I call for the regulation of technological development through prudence, prudence exercised in two main forms: foresight and vigilance. Foresight requires, among other things, a rigorous effort to forecast; vigilance demands debate and the creation of surveillance organizations.

IKEDA • This makes me think of several incidents that occurred in Japan several years ago, and of the unthinkable reactions of some of the scientists involved. Cases of organic-mercury poisoning and asthma were cropping up all over Japan. To protect the industry responsible for the pollution causing the problems, some scientists deliberately concealed or fraudulently concocted important data, even though people were suffering serious consequences. Something similar happened later in a suit involving the use of HIV-contaminated blood products for the treatment of hemophiliacs.

Why do such things happen? Perhaps, carried away by a sense of their own importance, the specialists take a narrow view of a situation and forget the ethical stance we justly expect of them. Perhaps desire for personal profit blinds them.

BOURGEAULT • In the global framework of savage competition, business and its engineers are more concerned with using advanced technology to produce more at lower costs than with considering risks. For their part, governments are more preoccupied with promoting immediate economic prosperity and preserving social order—more pragmatically still, with ensuring their own re-election—than with guarding the security of the citizens of tomorrow and the next day. When disaster threatens, or even in the midst of a catastrophe, governments tend to simply reassure us.

Somewhere between blessed tranquility and exhausting militancy, and generally distanced from decision-making, the ordinary citizenry lives in ignorance of the true state of affairs, an ignorance that cannot be dispelled by the divergent opinions of various experts. Facing the possibility of a major accident or catastrophe, the citizen is condemned to impotence in advance and knows that they are helpless. And when the worst happens—ostensibly unexpectedly, in spite of "warning shots"—the dilution of responsibility neutralizes efforts and leads to inertia.

As you point out, we saw this in the contaminated blood scandals that struck several countries. While discussions dragged on, no restrictions were put on blood transfusions that turned out to be catastrophic for hemophiliacs who, in the hundreds and thousands, became victims of HIV and its ravages.

IKEDA • Essentially no one can escape ethical responsibility for scientific technology. Moved by a sense of shared responsibility, ordinary citizens must find ways to take part in democratic discussions on science and technology.

Technological information is widely available. Specialized technicians and research workers must no longer monopolize technoscientific knowledge. As we mentioned in our discussion of cancer, doctor-patient relations are changing. The idea of informed consent is steadily gaining ground. And patients are being much more selective in choosing who will treat them and where. I applaud the tendency for the general public to demand a voice in the choice of specialists and to become actively involved in acquiring technical know-how.

SIMARD • I agree with you, Mr. Ikeda. In a lecture entitled "Technology and Responsibility," I argued that the choice of technology and specialized expertise is as much a social and political question as a technical one, and that it must therefore be submitted to broad democratic debate.

IKEDA • By leaving important issues entirely up to the specialists of various fields, ordinary citizens are relinquishing their right to make their own opinions heard. It is almost as if the resignation of ordinary citizens invites specialists and scientists to assume control.

BOURGEAULT • Ensuring wide participation in decisions that affect the life of all citizens is both a sign and a pledge of the democratic health of a society.

IKEDA • A few years ago, in my conversations with the late Linus Pauling (1901–94), he vigorously warned against the control exerted by scientists. If there is a way to avoid having science betray humanity rather than helping us, I think it lies in the hands of the scientists themselves. They must embrace steadfast ethical views. To cultivate a broadly human position, they must stay in touch with ordinary people and then deliberate on their way of life and on their rules of conduct from a broadly human consideration. In this connection, philosophy and religion have great significance.

The end of a common Western philosophical and scientific culture

BOURGEAULT • Over a long period in the West, ethics—or, more generally, philosophy—and scientific research developed within what I would call a common culture. Consonance, cooperation, even complicity took place between them in a kind of ceaseless, mutual fertilization. On the basis of a fundamentally shared vision of the world, philosophers, theologians, and jurists set their minds to the explanation of the demands of natural law and natural rights. For their part, doctors and physicians strove to discover and understand the laws of natural physics and physiology. They insisted that, far from being their own inventions, these laws were absolutely elemental, active in reality, and endowed with universal and perennial value or efficacy. Immanuel Kant could admiringly compare two different orders of equally immutable laws: the eternal movement of the stars in the sky and the moral law inscribed in the human heart.

IKEDA • At that time, science was respectful toward nature and humble before the mystery of the universe. Wonderful things near at hand, though beyond human ken, provided the common wellspring of both science and philosophy.

But as science advanced, the number of things explainable by means of its unique analytical methods grew to the point where science seemed omnipotent, able to answer all questions and solve all problems.

BOURGEAULT • Later, both philosophy and science became more sensitive to subjective and situational dimensions—to relative and relativizing dimensions. They became as sensitive to perceptions and conceptions as to scientific and philosophic practices. Later still, awareness of socio-cultural conditioning of both visions and practices intensified. The alliance between philosophy and science was not severed by these developments, however, not in the way it seems to be now in the wake of the collapse of their common cultural universe.

IKEDA • Still, the sense of awe for the unfathomable was lost. People became incapable of imagining a universal foundation transcending time and space. Although the change meant liberation from a dogmatic world view centered on an unconditionally absolute god, it also destroyed the common foundation between the human self and the world, leaving humanity adrift.

BOURGEAULT • Today, philosophy and ethics on the one hand and science and professional practices on the other belong in two different cultural worlds. This is no doubt why, in spite of the proliferation of professional ethics, there is no established coherence. This is also the reason why, in spite of innumerable seminars and symposia, ethics remains impotent to orient and define technoscientific practices.

IKEDA • Liberation from the old world view generated great value for humanity by allowing science to expand its areas of operation and become diversely productive. To their contemporaries, the great post-Renaissance scientific achievers—like Galileo and Copernicus—seemed to think and act boldly and to demonstrate no fear of God. They must have had profound faith in human possibilities. Their ideas and their works were inspired by the philosophic foundation of humanism.

Scientists today, on the other hand, having razed that foundation, concentrate solely on technological aspects, causing all kinds of conflicts in the process.

The new confluence of technoscience and ethics

BOURGEAULT • Modern science no longer has the contemplative character of classical science. As Ilya Prigogine and Isabelle Stengers observed twenty years ago, the distinguishing character of modern science is a confluence of technique and theory, a systematic alliance between the ambition to shape the world and the ambition to understand it.[7] The secular alliance between a philosophy oriented toward wisdom and a "theoretical" science, founded on observation, has been broken. The same break affected the complicity between natural-law morality and the scientific process that probed the laws of a nature it could not comprehend, influence or control. Jean Ladrière (1921–) wrote that, having formed an alliance not with philosophy, but with technology, science has become "operative."[8]

IKEDA • Since the old philosophical foundation is no longer equal to the task, we must create a broader, deeper philosophical basis on which to build the colossal edifice of modern science. We require a full overview of the expansive and ever-receding horizon of science and a compass to set the course that humanity must follow in the future.

BOURGEAULT • In contemporary societies, technological development gives rise to new philosophical and ethical questions that pose a major challenge. From the standpoint of modern science, traditional morality is pre-scientific. The ethics of our time—although not necessarily a science itself—cannot skimp on rigorous analyses and scientific studies of reality if it intends to guide and orient human action. Science has long been subject to ethics. Today ethics must build itself either on or with science, which is inevitably linked to technology. Technology has modified the cultural universe. Philosophy and especially ethics must take this into consideration.

A definitely short-sighted, simplistic view positions technology in the amoral economy of instruments and means. But technological

---

7. Ilya Prigogine and Isabelle Stengers. *Order out of Chaos: Man's New Dialogue with Nature.* New York: Random House. 1984.

8. Jean Ladrière. *The Challenge Presented to Cultures by Science and Technology.* Paris: UNESCO. 1977.

development carries questions of a philosophical or purely ethical order. Technological developments of the past decades make ethical judgment both necessary and urgent. Should human beings do things simply because we *can* do them? Is it right to do so? Is it advantageous? If so, to whom? And who will ultimately answer these questions and make the choices that naturally follow?

Today the new confluence of science and technology with philosophy and ethics must reflect on these fundamental, yet practical, questions.

IKEDA • How right you are! The fundamental and the practical, the universal and the specific are essentially inseparable. Buddhism teaches that truth resides both in the universal—eternal and immutable life—and the specific—the inexhaustible wisdom that adapts to changing circumstances.

The mystical and eternal objects of philosophy and ethics do not manifest themselves apart from the concrete and specific details revealed by analytical science and technology. The Buddhist concept of the true aspect of all phenomena (*shoho-jisso*) asserts that truth or ultimate reality is inherent in all things and is in no way different from them.

Buddhism also teaches that the ability to grasp the true aspect of all phenomena varies from era to era and society to society. The Buddhist is expected to investigate both the universal and the particular, repeatedly. In this way, understanding is both deepened and carried to higher levels.

The bodhisattva way consists in the search for eternal truth. Indeed, the word bodhisattva means a seeker after ultimate wisdom.

5. Century of Life

The joy of learning: Contributing to society

IKEDA • We have arrived at last at our final topic. We would like to conclude our exchange by discussing the development of individuals who can make the twenty-first century radiant, a century dedicated to the respect for the dignity of life. The aging of society will be an important issue in the coming century. In industrialized nations where the populations are already greying, great attention is being paid to the quality and meaning of life.

Each of us has the responsibility to continue developing our potential throughout our lives, even after we finish our formal education and venture into the world. The Russian writer and founder of Moscow State University, Mikhail V. Lomonosov (1711–65), wrote that learning cultivates the young and delights the old. Without learning, human beings are not truly human.

SIMARD · I think that for students, education is the joy of learning and the possibility of thinking for themselves.

IKEDA · Yes, the joy of improving and standing on their own . . . that's it, isn't it?

SIMARD · Once discovered, that joy remains a treasure for life. Essentially, education consists in teaching the need to learn constantly throughout life. That is more important than transmitting accumulated knowledge.

BOURGEAULT · A very interesting book published a few years ago argued that, without the joy of learning, constant study would be like life imprisonment.

IKEDA · There is a lot of truth in that.

BOURGEAULT · How can we avoid turning lifelong education into perpetual imprisonment? This is a fascinating question. First, the learner must discover that the true joy of learning is experienced not by dodging obstacles and difficulties, but by surmounting them.

IKEDA · The Buddhist scriptures teach that birth and death are one with nirvana. We must challenge and overcome the sufferings of birth and death to reach a state of true happiness called nirvana. Likewise, in education, the learner cannot experience the joy of learning without first experiencing difficulty and overcoming it.

In other words, we must study for the benefit of society and in the service of others. This, too, evokes both joy and new discoveries. I believe this is indisputable.

SIMARD • Fairly early on, we at the University of Montreal undertook a project of developing objectives and orientations for lifelong education in a perspective close to Dr. Bourgeault's ideas.

The content of lifelong-education programs has changed over time. One of our programs—unique in its field—is directed toward people already in the labor market. In our era of rapid social and technological mutation, workers are constantly being pressured to improve their skills and acquire new knowledge. Our Faculty of Continuing Education provides various courses designed to improve professional skills.

In a highly industrialized country like Canada, where the numbers of professionals and well-educated people are constantly growing and where cultural diversity and the volume of information continually increase, it is almost imperative to continue training in one way or another. Otherwise the labor market quickly leaves you behind. Today, most people take for granted the need to devote themselves to some kind of continuing education. Of course, we also have many programs in liberal arts and the artistic and literary activities people engage in mainly for pleasure.

IKEDA • It is inspiring to hear how your university seeks to adapt its continuing education programs to the changing needs of society and simultaneously help people continue their training, moved by the joy of learning and the hopes of contributing to society. At Soka University, we have established a correspondence program that offers courses to anyone who wishes to apply.

SIMARD • Yes, I know a little about Soka University's correspondence program.

IKEDA • The tombstone of Leonardo da Vinci (1452–1519) reads: A full life is long, a full day brings sound sleep, and an accomplished life brings a tranquil death. Constant learning and improvement vastly enrich life. My mentor, Josei Toda, used to tell us, "How you end your life is what counts. No matter what may have happened over the years, the true winner is happy and fulfilled to the very end. I hope my twilight years will be like a glorious sunset." My wish for people in the twenty-first century is that, right to the end, their lives will shine like the sun.

Appreciating differences polishes the conscience of the world citizen

SIMARD • The twenty-first century is going to be the age of information. How should universities respond to the needs created by computers and information technology? This is a new issue. Currently, new training programs are being developed on the basis of leading-edge telecommunications and electronic data transmission. One of them is the intelligent self-instruction system. What do you think about these new programs, Mr. Ikeda?

IKEDA • Study methods must change in the information society. Soka University students and faculty members can conduct Internet searches for information all over the world. At Soka Women's Junior College, English is taught over the Internet. Knowledge is no longer necessarily transmitted from individual to individual. On our own initiative we can seek out and obtain information from sources all over the world, study and analyze the data we select and even "chat" with people in distant lands. We have entered an era when we can study together and illuminate each other's minds on a global scale. Costa Rican President Jose Maria Figueres Olsen (1954–) once told me that he hoped to educate his people to be bilingual and computer literate and to serve society.

SIMARD • Mastery of one's native language is essential for both the acquisition and the transmission of knowledge. This is an indispensable condition for a rich, diversified, autonomous intellectual life. Coherent thought is impossible without coherent, correctly structured language. Neither perception nor oral or written expression of the universe is possible without mastery of a language that contributes to the simultaneous shaping and expression of the individual. Learning a second or third language is much more than acquiring additional communication tools, although of course these are indispensable in our North-South American context or your Asiatic context. Language learning is the key to modes of thought and expression we cannot afford to remain strangers with.

People of the twenty-first century must master other, non-linguistic languages as well. No field of knowledge can bypass the language of mathematics, not to mention the informational idiom that has become its necessary counterpart. Can we dispense with minimal knowledge of these two forms of language if we wish to go even a little deeper into any of the basic disciplines?

And what is to be said of artistic forms of expression? Should not a cultivated person be in a position to read these forms, too—the literary, the pictorial, the musical and the tactile? Indeed, it is not enough for our societies to make progress on the technological plane. They must also participate in a more human world cognizant of similar breakthroughs on the levels of conscience, knowledge, and expression of all human dimensions.

IKEDA · That is quite true. Computer skills and foreign languages have given people the means to appreciate diverse cultures and ethnic traditions, and can help inculcate an awareness of world-citizenship. True citizens of the world know how to understand the hearts and minds of people who live elsewhere. They have a perceptive intuition that enables them to cooperate and share with others.

SIMARD · We are witnessing the intensification of economic and political ties and international interdependence. Students must learn to be tolerant of cultural diversity and to think from a global vantage point. Awareness that one's own existence is always bound to the existence of others on the planet engenders an acute sense of responsibility. As more and more people become citizens of the world, the shock of coming into contact with other societies and traditions will become trivial.

IKEDA · It seems to me that an authentic feeling of world citizenship will naturally arise from the meeting of diverse traditions. Aware of their differences, people will make an effort to discover what they have in common and what they agree on. To nourish this cosmopolitan awakening, people must welcome diversity, allow others to be different and recognize the right to be different.

Nichiren Daishonin once said: "When one faces a mirror and bows, the image in the mirror bows back."[9] Respecting the wonder of the lives of a diverse array of other people reflects dignity on our own

9. *Gosho Zenshu.* 769.

lives. Showing respect for differences is the best way to develop our own individualities.

Four vows of bodhisattvas

BOURGEAULT • Encountering *others*—different from us and considered odd because they are strangers—poses a serious problem in today's societies, with their plurality of origins, traditions, and cultures. The *other* is no longer in some more or less remote place, but here, close at hand.

We often hear it said that regular association cultivates better understanding, making it easier for us to live together with *others*. But experience shows that this is not always the case. Association sometimes highlights divergences of opinion and convictions, evoking fear and either retreat or aggression, rather than comprehension and mutual aid. If, even unconsciously, we consider ourselves the measure and definition of Man, we condemn *others* for being different from us, without even considering that, for them, we ourselves are the *others*. It is therefore important to acknowledge the diversity of reality—especially of human beings and of ways of being human—more than the differences that always establish ourselves as models and gauges.

On the basis of ideas expressed by Tzvétan Todorov (1939–) in *On Human Diversity: Nationalism, Racism and Exoticism in French Thought*,[10] I distinguish three kinds of attitudes toward differences perceived in social diversity: (1) feelings of anxiety that lead to, if not always rejection, at least a refusal to interact with the *others* and their subsequent ostracism and marginalization; (2) fascination with the exotic that leads to an exaggeration of differences and ultimately inhibits true exchange; and (3) willingness to tolerate a disturbing encounter because it leads to a joint revision of ways of thinking and acting, of negotiating arrangements, and exchanging for the sake of new social relationships.

IKEDA • The process of exchange you have just described has a lot in common with the bodhisattva way.

---

10. Tzvétan Todorov. *On Human Diversity: Nationalism, Racism and Exoticism in French Thought*. Tr. Catherine Porter. Cambridge: Harvard University Press. 1993.

In examining the goals of education, Tsunesaburo Makiguchi said
that priority must be given to the way people develop a sense of
purpose in life, because our reasons for living and our reasons for
studying are one and the same thing. The basic posture of Buddhism—especially Mahayana Buddhism—is to constantly struggle to
make life richer and more fruitful. The four vows a bodhisattva makes
when first resolving to embark upon Buddhist practice represent the
purpose of Buddhist study, that is, the goals of a bodhisattva's life.

The first vow is to save all sentient beings, in other words, to make
all people happy. Nichiren Daishonin considered this the most important of the vows since the fundamental goal of Buddhism is happiness
for the self and for others.[11] This corresponds to a sense of responsibility for the whole.

The second vow, to eradicate countless delusions, expresses determination to triumph over the greed, anger, and folly that obscure the
lesser ego. It is connected with the way of life that, freed from egoism, transcends suffering and manifests wisdom with courage and
unshakable ideals.

The third vow is to master innumerable Buddhist teachings that
encompass all laws and all phenomena. We can interpret this as an
exhortation to respect and study the vast stores of knowledge humans
have collected and the diverse cultures we have created, and to continue our search for the truth for the sake of freeing humanity from
suffering.

The fourth vow is to attain supreme enlightenment. This is a vow
to persist unflaggingly in seeking human perfection. This last vow is
related to the idea of continuing education we were speaking of earlier.

These four fundamental vows outline a way of life dedicated to
self-improvement and the well-being of others. I consider the goals of
the vows essential conditions to the truly cosmopolitan world citizen.

Inventing new views of humanity and the world

BOURGEAULT • But I do not believe we can find a recipe for a perfect
citizen in any tradition of religious inspiration. Returning to certitudes,

11. "After all, you must regard the vow to save innumerable living beings as foremost among the four universal vows [of bodhisattvas.]" *Gosho Zenshu*. 846.

it seems to me that religions tend to discredit—even reject—people who break with their dogmas. Today we need visions of the world that take diversity into consideration. A synopsis of history shows that religions have given moral support to too many wars—sometimes called holy wars—and to too many other forms of violence. Even today, devastating religious and ethnic wars dramatically bear witness to the weight of that heritage.

IKEDA • It is a deplorable state of affairs, indeed. What we need now is religion that serves the people, not the inverse. The minimal condition for a religion of the twenty-first century is that it be open to humanity and the world.

BOURGEAULT • I think it is possible to establish ethics and a way of life free of pre-established visions of humanity and the world. More precisely, I mean ethics with no consensus that defines in advance humanity, the world and the meaning of life and plots a course to the good. I believe that such ethics are necessary, because technology now permits such decisive action that the vision of humanity and the world that is likely to orient our choices and actions is no longer behind but before us.

We now perceive humanity and the world not as definitively constituted, given realities, but as things in the process of being formed. Since we have the power to do so, we can decide what kind of humanity we will be tomorrow and take requisite measures to preserve the quality of the environment our descendants will live in. Life and quality of life have become our responsibility.

The essential landmarks of ethical behavior are no longer those that imposed a pre-established vision of humanity and the world yesterday. Just as the ancient Hebrews journeying toward an inaccessible land discovered the meaning of their destiny along the way, similarly, working together, we can shape and live the new adventure of human life entrusted to our hands and to our responsibility.

IKEDA • I agree with you wholeheartedly. The twenty-first century must be a century "of the people, by the people, and for the people."

BOURGEAULT • You might say that the solidarity born of encounters and discussions with others and lived in the exercise of shared responsibility is itself religious insofar as it reconnects humans to humans and to their environment, in the global Buddhist perspective to which you have referred. But I see no need for humans to search outside of—or above—themselves for legitimization of their existence, as has been done in Western religious traditions. No more is there a need to seek it within, in something deeper than ourselves where we commune with an inclusive spiritual element.

A certain Christian spirituality advocates the love of human beings "for the love of God." It seems to me that human beings are worthy of being loved for themselves, for what they are: fragile and transitory travelling companions, by day and by night. It is unnecessary to transcend man in order to love man and all human beings, male or female, with whom we can simply experience the joys and pains of a common odyssey.

IKEDA • What you say reminds me of the bodhisattva compassion. When ordinary human beings share the pains and joys of the continuing search for happiness, their acts are compassionate. As a Buddhist, I see something infinitely noble in this difficult under-taking. It reveals the dignity of humanity. Certainly the individual human being is fragile and ephemeral. But there is greatness in the individual, too. Surely we may be permitted to designate dignified human affection as the compassion of the Buddha or the love of God. Whatever we call it, however, I hope it will guide us in the struggle to make this a radiant century of life.

Why Buddhism became a world religion

SIMARD • Since its emergence, in the fifth century BCE, the Buddhist system of thought and belief has exerted an enormous influence on humanity and has spread to many parts of the world. Why? What factors account for this development?

IKEDA • A number of explanations come to mind. Buddhism became a world religion partly because it broaches a fundamental issue experi-enced by all people: salvation from suffering.

SIMARD • Are you referring to the four sufferings of birth, aging, sick-ness, and death that you mentioned earlier?

IKEDA · Yes, but Buddhism in fact lists eight sufferings, the four you mention plus the suffering of having to part from those we love, the suffering of having to meet those we hate, the suffering of being unable to obtain what we desire, and the suffering arising from the five components of mind and body.

Shakyamuni's challenge of these sufferings and his certitude that it is possible to overcome them are the starting point of Buddhism. He renounced the rank of prince and gave up secular life to pursue the life of a wandering monk. For years he submitted to a life of rigorous discipline and asceticism. Finally he meditated and attained enlightenment, seated under the bodhi tree. Enlightenment means awakening to the ultimate law of the universe. This law is universal because it throbs in the depths of human lives and in all living beings.

The second reason Buddhism has become a universal religion is because Shakyamuni attained enlightenment and perceived the universal law. Because the law transcends race, ethnicity, nationality and culture, the Buddha's teachings spread within his country and elsewhere, regardless of barriers that divide the phenomenal world.

Thirdly, Shakyamuni awakened to a law that, far from being a dry abstraction, radiates compassion and wisdom on everything in the universe, including humans. Buddhist wisdom has inspired the prodigious works of countless scholars working together to develop an extremely refined philosophical system.

Among them let me mention Nagarjuna, a Mahayana scholar from Southern India who lived in the second and third centuries BCE, famous for his classification of the doctrine of non-substantiality or latency; Vasubandhu, an Indian scholar from the fourth and fifth centuries BCE, widely known for his Consciousness-Only teaching; and China's T'ien-t'ai or Chih-i (538–597) who propounded the doctrine of Three Thousand Realms in a Single Life Moment on the basis of the *Lotus Sutra*. The complex system and rigorous logic of these subtle teachings appealed to people and became the core of their faith.

SIMARD · I assume you are referring to the concept of Buddha nature and to the doctrine of causation which you discussed earlier.

IKEDA · Yes. Furthermore, since Buddhist wisdom is rooted in the power of compassion at the core of the universe, the bodhisattva way of altruistic service and striving to eliminate the suffering of others inevitably evolved from it. To practice the bodhisattva way is to resolutely reject violence and support non-violence. And this is the fourth reason for the worldwide spread of Buddhism.

BOURGEAULT • I first encountered Buddhism and its traditions while making a somewhat fragmentary study of the history of religions. I was concentrating on Western history and I was struck by the fact that conflicts between religions often led to wars between nations. In many cases, the wars arose from other causes, but as tensions mounted, religions became involved. At least this has often happened in the West. I suspect similar phenomena have occurred in the history of Buddhism.

IKEDA • Your suspicion points directly to the issue of non-violence. Let me give an example. In the third century BCE, the Indian King Ashoka began his reign as a tyrant but later resolved to reflect the spirit of Shakyamuni in politics. The change occurred in 259 BCE, when he had just conquered a district known as Kalinga. Seeing the misery of the conquered people, his eyes were opened to his own cruelty. He began to develop a fervent Buddhist faith. He renounced warfare and conquest and instituted a reign of peace, sending emissaries of the Buddhist Law to all the neighboring states and territories.

Under his tolerant policies, diverse cultures flourished. Though a Buddhist himself, he guaranteed the religious freedom of the Jainists, the Brahmans and other ethnic groups.

This tolerance, combined with its non-violence, is the fifth reason why Buddhism has spread far and wide. The Buddhist spirit of tolerance has cultivated respect for human rights and human dignity and diversity, thereby encouraging cultural creativity. These attitudes helped it find a place in an already sophisticated Chinese civilization and in the rich cultures of other Asian regions.

Compromises with power

BOURGEAULT • Our discussions have helped me understand Buddhism a little better. At the risk of being simplistic and uncritical, I would summarize as follows: On one side—with Buddhism and more generally with what we call oriental wisdom—we find interiorized contemplation, non-violence and tolerance, solidarity and compassion. On the other, the will to control the world through actions stimulating technoscientific development, free enterprise and competition, and—when need be—war. But hasn't the Orient also known war and violence? And haven't religion in general and Buddhism in particular been involved in disputes? Haven't non-violence, tolerance, and even the duty of compassion been used—at least in certain instances—as instruments of domination?

IKEDA • As you have suggested, the Buddhist spirit of tolerance has sometimes lost substance and become synonymous with acceptance of the status quo. This tendency has led to stagnation, deterioration, and—worse—to compromise with the reigning authorities.

In some instances, the state made use of Buddhism; in others, Buddhism made use of the power of the state. Collusion with power naturally led to the deterioration of Buddhism as a system of thoughts and beliefs, and to the degradation and corruption of the priesthood. The connivance of certain Buddhist groups with the military government in Japan in the middle of the twentieth century is a good example in recent history. Some sects even gave active moral support to Japanese participation in the Second World War. One notable exception: Tsunesaburo Makiguchi, founding president of the Soka Gakkai, was ferociously opposed to Japanese militarism. As you probably know, these views led him to die in prison at the age of 73.

BOURGEAULT • Yes, I know the terrible circumstances of his death.

IKEDA • In my dialogue with Dr. Johan Galtung (1930–), founder director of the Peace Research Institute of Oslo (PRIO),[12] he said that, unlike Christianity or Islam, Buddhism presents the qualities of tolerance and diversity essential to a philosophy of peace. On the other hand, he added, precisely because of its tolerance, Buddhism has tended to accept such examples of structural violence as tyranny, the oppression of the poor, and human-rights violations.

BOURGEAULT • Christianity has been guilty of similar weaknesses and perversions. I appreciate your willingness to reveal them in Buddhism.

---

12. Johan Galtung and Daisaku Ikeda. *Choose Peace: A Dialogue.* London: Pluto Press. 1995.

Nichiren Buddhism and Shakyamuni Buddhism

SIMARD • Buddhism has spread to many parts of the world and of course has had enormous influence in Japan. I believe Japan became a Buddhist country in ancient times.

IKEDA • Yes, Buddhism was officially introduced to Japan by the regent Prince Shotoku (574–622).

SIMARD • Then in the thirteenth century Japanese Buddhism underwent a reformation. One of the best known reformers was Nichiren Daishonin, as I understand it. What was Nichiren Buddhism like in the thirteenth century?

IKEDA • As Buddhist history makes clear, attaining enlightenment to the universal law through one's own efforts, as Shakyamuni did, demands extremely strict discipline. After Shakyamuni's death, Buddhism lapsed into complicated, speculative philosophy that grew too abstruse for ordinary people. To bridge the gap, Mahayana Buddhism called for a return to the original spirit of Shakyamuni and encouraged the bodhisattva ideal. But, as time passed, Mahayana Buddhism burdened itself with many levels of practice and complex interpretations too demanding for all but scholarly monks and zealots. Even the T'ien-t'ai system developed a complex set of observances that took monks over a decade to perfect.

Nichiren Daishonin felt that people should be able to manifest their inherent Buddha nature in the context of daily life. To help them do this, he created a mandala, an object of worship on which he inscribed the law of the universe. In doing so, he showed how all people can manifest their Buddha nature and overcome the four sufferings. In this way, Nichiren established a Buddhist practice that is truly for the people.

SIMARD • What are the specific differences between Nichiren Buddhism and historic Shakyamuni Buddhism?

IKEDA • Over time, Shakyamuni's Buddhism lost ground and compromised with political leaders, becoming an instrument of control. Its collusion with political authority led to the oppression of the masses. Originally, the Buddhist spirit of tolerance had nothing to do with compromise or condoning political injustice. The true nature of its tolerance was to struggle against oppression by the powerful.

Buddhist tolerance is synonymous with compassion. True compassion fights against power that inflicts sorrow on ordinary people. The word "tolerance" also qualifies this combative spirit. "Compassion" in the Buddhist sense means both empathy for the people's suffering and commitment to help them overcome it. Empathy for the suffering of others, or sharing that suffering, can be compared with motherly love. Fatherly love symbolizes action to remove the causes of suffering. Mother's love is unconditional and all-embracing. Father's love discriminates between the just and the unjust and fights sternly against evil. Shakyamuni's Buddhism became more inclined to motherly love, so to speak, and let slide the fatherly aspect of combatting evil. Since it combines both maternal and paternal love, the Buddhism of Nichiren Daishonin offers a just balance of tenderness and rigor. The fatherly side is expressed in the incessant fight against injustice and against the forces that oppress the people and provoke misery.

SIMARD · What attitude did Nichiren Buddhism take toward the ruling authorities of his time?

IKEDA · Whenever it was necessary, Nichiren remonstrated with the government.

In thirteenth century Japan, all established sects of Buddhism had been incorporated into the political structure and therefore supported the authorities, not the people. Nichiren stayed resolutely on the side of the people, never withdrawing from the struggle. He himself wrote, "The varied sufferings of all living beings—all these Nichiren himself accepts as his own sufferings!"[13] He also taught, "In the final analysis, unless we succeed in demonstrating that this teaching is supreme, these disasters will continue unabated."[14] His courageous resistance is a remarkable change in the history of Buddhism.

To summarize, true Buddhist compassion is at once like maternal love, sympathizing with and embracing the sufferings of all sentient beings, and like paternal love, determined to fight on to the end until suffering has been eliminated and true serenity established. Of course,

13. *Gosho Zenshu.* 758.
14. *The Writings of Nichiren Daishonin.* 1114.

the terms "benevolent mother" and "strict father" in this context are metaphorical references to the virtues of the Buddha and do not pertain to real human family relations.

Buddhism for peace

SIMARD • What was Japan like at the time when Nichiren Buddhism set out to achieve social reform?

IKEDA • Established Buddhism was out of phase with social realities and bred only hypocrisy. Compromising with political authority, the priesthood distorted the fundamental teachings. A tyrannical government that Buddhist groups not only failed to put in check, but actively supported—such was the reality that Nichiren Daishonin wanted to change with his Buddhist reform. Nichiren Daishonin insisted that Buddhism must always contribute to peace and become a useful practical teaching for society. This is the heart of his treatise *On Establishing the Correct Teaching for the Peace of the Land*.

BOURGEAULT • I remember your earlier explanation of it.

IKEDA • Yes, I already explained the persecutions Nichiren faced for this treatise and his courageous struggle with the authorities. The *Lotus Sutra* teaches that the ideal realm is not located in some distant place isolated from actual society.[15] The ordinary world and the "Land of Eternally Tranquil Light" where the Buddha resides are one. This means that the harsh world of reality is the place where we must create an ideal of peace and prosperity, wisdom and boundless compassion.

Nichiren Daishonin proposed the ideas in *On Establishing the Correct Teaching* in order to transform Japan—and the whole world— into the ideal realm described in the *Lotus Sutra*. In other words, he wanted to create a Buddha land founded on the fundamental law of the universe, a treasure land of peace where human rights would be respected and humanity could live in harmonious coexistence with the natural environment.

Having inherited the spirit and the ideals of Nichiren, the young people of SGI are also heirs to the thoughts Josei Toda expressed in

15. *The Lotus Sutra*. 225.

1957, when he proclaimed the use of nuclear weapons to be an absolute evil. The use of weapons of mass destruction could wipe humanity—and how much more!—off the face of the earth. Struggling against this evil is the bodhisattva way of our time. The youth of SGI are working actively today, the world over, to put Toda's exhortation into practice and campaign for the abolition of nuclear weapons, for peace, for human rights and for environmental conservation.

Buddhism in daily life

SIMARD • What difference does practicing the Buddhism of Nichiren instead of the Buddhism of Shakyamuni make in daily life?

IKEDA • It is significant that, whereas Shakyamuni was born a prince, Nichiren Daishonin was the son of a fisherman. Shakyamuni's Buddhism tended to compromise with authority and condone oppression. At the same time, it could flee from secular authority in the pursuit of personal tranquility far from society.

In contrast, the Buddhism of Nichiren Daishonin is integrated with the lives of the ordinary people. It strives to work with others to create a realm of imperishable happiness. Nichiren Daishonin said, "A person of wisdom is not one who practices Buddhism apart from worldly affairs but, rather, one who thoroughly understands the principles by which the world is governed."[16] In other words, it is our mission to apply the fundamental law of the universe in our daily life when we are involved in politics, economics, learning, culture, science, and so on.

We must neither be defeated by nor try to evade the sufferings of reality. Instead of fleeing from them, we must challenge the four sufferings head-on and look on them as opportunities for self-discipline. At the same time, we must empathize with the sufferings of others and cooperate with them in the battle to turn sorrow into happiness. Furthermore we must take the campaign to overcome the four sufferings into workplaces, family circles, neighborhoods, and regional societies in all parts of the world and into all cultural spheres and races.

16. *The Writings of Nichiren Daishonin.* 1466.

In some cases, the struggle will take the form of the battle for human rights against oppressive officials or corrupt clergymen. The Buddhism of Nichiren Daishonin makes clear that the world of suffering and the "Land of Eternally Tranquil Light" are one and the same; this world of both possibilities is right here on earth. It admonishes us to realize this ideal not in some distant never-never land, but here and now.

SIMARD · I begin to see Buddhism as a solid philosophy for the reformation of our world.

IKEDA · One of Makiguchi's education reforms proposed including a "Hometown Course" in the elementary cycle, because the places where children are born and raised are their starting points in life. From there, exchanges, dialogues, and an expanding network of solidarity would foster awareness of membership in a global citizenry.

BOURGEAULT · I, too, believe that without a solid awareness of one's immediate local community environment, the concept of global citizen is only a hollow formula. Owing to the push of globalization, the larger world encroaches more and more on local communities. Each place is going to be increasingly attached to all other places. Becoming a citizen of the world does not require us to leave our native communities. On the contrary, it is first necessary to accept membership in our home place and recognize the specific culture or unique way of thinking and behaving that we have inherited. Then we must enter into dialogue and debate with others, share with them, and—if I may put it this way—try to remake the whole world.

IKEDA · You are right. A citizen of the world is not some special kind of person, but merely a person with an open mind and with compassion, courage, and wisdom.

SIMARD · The University of Montreal has devoted serious effort to internationalizing its programs, developing new teaching and training methods, and improving its foreign-language programs. It also proposes dynamic student exchange programs, staff instruction, and research with other universities throughout the world, including, of course, Soka University.

IKEDA · You are making precious contributions to stimulating awareness of world citizenship. Having concluded agreements with universities all over the world, including the University of Montreal, Soka University engages in a lively program of student and faculty exchanges. I hope our two institutions can continue to work together to provide scientific and cultural information and global contacts to as many people as possible. I further hope that we can train and send abroad young citizens of the world who will do their utmost for the peace and prosperity of humankind.

Postscript

A<small>T THE CONCLUSION</small> of our "trialogue" on human life and health, it is, of course, impossible to tally up the results of this encounter between medical science and the evolution of medical practices, on one side, and ethical concern for the future of individuals, whole societies and the human race, on the other. The outcome, obviously, is humble. We have blazed some trails for thought, and perhaps for action. We have discussed some questions that we deem crucial and urgent, questions about life and death, health and illness. Most of all, we have discussed the meaning we can give to our own irremediably mortal lives—fragile, limited, and vulnerable to illness—and our constant struggle, our incessant search for balance.

Discussions of life and health usually remain well within the limits of the biomedical domain—scientific, technological, and professional. In our discussions, however, we transcended those limits to include the anthropological, social, and political dimensions too often ignored. We explored social ethics and global issues. At the heart of problems linked to globalization—liberalization of financial policies, rationalization, relocation of multinational production to countries with lax laws and more easily exploitable labor, deregulation of an increasingly global market—problems that lead to social upheaval and political restructuring, lie the basic questions of life and death, the question of the health of individuals, societies and humankind in general. These are the very things that have produced humankind, and it is their future that we have discussed. Today's actions determine what kind of people we will be tomorrow.

The current dynamic of globalization is also nourished, however, by intercultural exchanges such as this dialogue. We have tried to break down the barriers between disciplines and cultures, not to quarrel, convince or win, but to learn from each other. To try to gain a better understanding of our ever-elusive reality.

We come away from these discussions with more questions than answers, but—we hope—with better-formulated questions. As we have said several times along the way, health is a ceaseless search for an equilibrium that is forever precarious. Likewise, our quest for meaning is constantly contradicted by life experiences that forever push us to renew the quest.

With our discussions over, we have each returned to our own path, the richer for the exchange. In reading this book, you too have participated in the discussion, and you too will return to your own unique path. We hope you find yourself enriched, more aware, and armed with a lucidity that boosts your momentum.

We hope that life will treat you well, and with this we extend both the wish and the invitation to work toward the creation of a world where life is good for the greatest possible number of people.

GUY BOURGEAULT
UNIVERSITY OF MONTREAL

Index

Also from Middleway Press

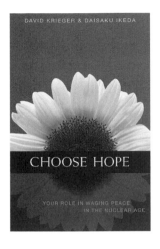

Choose Hope: Your Role in Waging Peace in the Nuclear Age, by David Krieger and Daisaku Ikeda
(ISBN 0-9674697-6-7; $23.95)
Silver Book of the Year Award, 2003, ForeWord Magazine

"In this nuclear age, when the future of humankind is imperiled by irrational strategies, it is imperative to restore sanity to our policies and hope to our destiny. Only a rational analysis of our problems can lead to their solution. This book is an example par excellence of a rational approach."
— Joseph Rotblat,
Nobel Peace Prize laureate

For the Sake of Peace: Seven Paths to Global Harmony, A Buddhist Perspective, by Daisaku Ikeda
Winner of the NAPRA Nautilus Award 2002 for Social Change

(ISBN 0-9674697-9-1; $14.00)

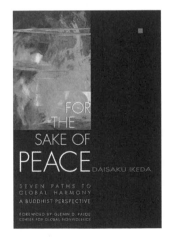

"At a time when we squander enormous amounts of human and environmental resources on the study of and preparation for making war, *For the Sake of Peace* stands as a primary text in the study and practice of making peace."
—NAPRA, Nautilus
Award citation

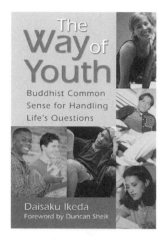

The Way of Youth: Buddhist Common Sense for Handling Life's Questions, by Daisaku Ikeda
(ISBN 0-9674697-0-8; $14.95)

Also available in Spanish
A la Manera de los Jovenés
(ISBN 0-9674697-3-2; $14.95)

"[This book] shows the reader how to flourish as a young person in the world today; how to build confidence and character in modern society; learn to live with respect for oneself and others; how to contribute to a positive, free and peaceful society; and find true personal happiness."
—Midwest Book Review

The Buddha in Your Mirror: Practical Buddhism and the Search for Self, by Woody Hochswender, Greg Martin and Ted Morino
(ISBN 0-9674697-8-3; $14.00)

Also available in Spanish
El Buda en Tu Espejo
(ISBN 0-9674697-7-5; $14.00)

"Like the Buddha, this book offers practical guidelines to overcome difficulties in everyday life and to be helpful to others. Readers will find these pages are like a helpful and supportive friend. I enthusiastically recommend it."
— Dr. David Chappell,
    editor of *Buddhist Peacework: Creating Cultures of Peace*

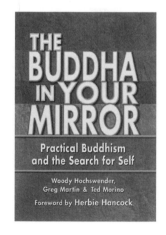

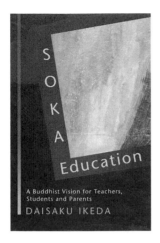

Soka Education: A Buddhist Vision for Teachers, Students and Parents, by Daisaku Ikeda
(ISBN 0-9674697-4-0; $23.95)

From the Japanese word meaning "to create value," this book presents a fresh spiritual perspective to question the ultimate purpose of education. Mixing American pragmatism with Buddhist philosophy, the goal of Soka education is the lifelong happiness of the learner.

"[Teachers] will be attracted to Soka and Ikeda's plea that educators bring heart and soul back to education."
—*Teacher* magazine

"Ikeda's practical perscription places students' needs first, empowers teachers, and serves as a framework for global citizenship."
—George David Miller, professor, Lewis University

Ask for Middleway Press books at your favorite neighborhood or on-line bookseller. Or visit www.middlewaypress.com.

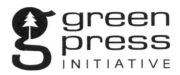

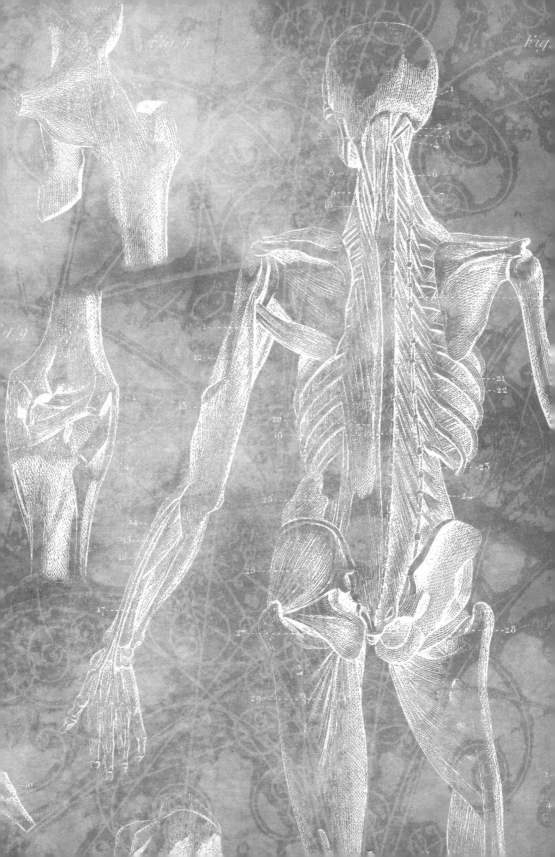